Gerrie Lim is the bestselling author of *Invisible Trade: High-Class Sex for Sale in Singapore*, his exposé of the escort business in Southeast Asia, *Invisible Trade II: Secret Lives and Sexual Intrigue in Singapore*, an exposé of sexual commerce in Singapore, and *In Lust We Trust: Adventures in Adult Cinema*, his memoir of a decade spent covering the erotica industry in Los Angeles, where he previously lived for fifteen years as a freelance writer contributing to *Billboard*, *Details*, *LA Style*, *LA Weekly*, *Penthouse*, *Playboy* and *The Wall Street Journal*. His most recent book, *Absolute Mayhem*, was co-written with pornstar Monica Mayhem and published in 2009, in Australian, American and French editions. This is his seventh book.

T0112046

OTHER BOOKS BY GERRIE LIM

Inside the Outsider
Invisible Trade
Invisible Trade II
Idol to Icon
In Lust We Trust
Absolute Mayhem

SEARCHING FOR ANNABEL CHONG

DEMYSTIFYING THE LEGEND OF SINGAPORE'S MOST FAMOUS PORNSTAR!

GERRIE LIM

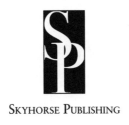

SKYHORSE PUBLISHING

Skyhorse Publishing books may be purchased in bulk at special discounts for sales promotion, corporate gifts, fund-raising, or educational purposes. Special editions can also be created to specifications. For details, contact the Special Sales Department, Skyhorse Publishing, 307 West 36th Street, 11th Floor, New York, NY 10018 or info@skyhorsepublishing.com.

Skyhorse® and Skyhorse Publishing® are registered trademarks of Skyhorse Publishing, Inc.®, a Delaware corporation.

Visit our website at www.skyhorsepublishing.com.

10 9 8 7 6 5 4 3 2 1

Library of Congress Cataloging-in-Publication Data is available on file.
ISBN: 978-1-61608-729-6

Printed in the United States of America

For P.H.

("Once more, with feeling")

CONTENTS

PROLOGUE: THE DEMON GODDESS   9

1   Persona Non Gratification   17
2   Messalina's Revenge   47
3   Double Trouble   72
4   Asian Fever   124
5   Chuck Palahniuk Loves Veronica Lake   151
6   Singapore Rebel   178
7   The Sand Mandala   192

POSTSCRIPT   209
ACKNOWLEDGMENTS   218

PROLOGUE

THE DEMON GODDESS

"I have nothing to declare but my genius."
Oscar Wilde, while passing through US Customs in 1881

Annabel Chong: her name rings a bell, even as it resonates like a bolt of lightning from the heavens.

Paul Theroux, the novelist and travel writer, describes her as "an amazing woman, a demon goddess out of a Chinese folk tale – the woman who dared to convert all her desires into reality – a fantasy to most men, and a sort of heroine to a lot of women, though they would probably not dare to admit it."

And why would they not dare admit it?

Because Annabel Chong remains the only famous pornstar from Singapore, a young woman who had put her home country on the map back in 1995 when she allowed herself to be filmed having sexual intercourse with a large group of men, each one waiting his turn, all done in the space of ten hours and for the posterity of home video. Reports said there were 251 men but there were actually only 70, though she was penetrated 251 times (with many of the men rejoining the end of the line for second and third rounds).

The film, *The World's Greatest Gangbang*, found itself under scrutiny in 1999, with the release of a documentary film about her life, *Sex: The Annabel Chong Story*, which premiered at the Sundance Film Festival in Park City, Utah. Not surprisingly, it garnered massive amounts of ink from both highbrow and lowbrow presses. Novelists like Bret Easton Ellis and Chuck Palahniuk have written about her (the former not so flatteringly, the latter more so). And in Singapore itself, she has long been regarded somewhere between a mythological figure and an urban legend.

But in actuality she did exist, though she wasn't always called Annabel Chong.

She was a precociously book-smart young girl, born Grace Quek in Singapore on May 22, 1972, who had gone to King's College London on a scholarship to study law. At age 21, she dropped out of law school and went to Los Angeles where she undertook courses in photography, art, and gender studies at the University of Southern California (the same university I attended, even though we were in different faculties and didn't know one another back then).

And then, her life changed forever. She joined the porn industry in 1994, at age 22, an event possibly triggered by something from her recent past. When she was living in

London, she had been gang-raped by some guys in an innercity housing estate after disembarking from a subway station.

That kind of thing only needs to happen to you once, for your life to change quite radically. The notion of being the girl in the gangbang probably first took root right there, on that fateful day.

In the documentary *Sex: The Annabel Chong Story*, made in 1998, she goes to London and revisits the actual scene of the rape, and it surely wasn't a segment of film spliced in accidentally. It was meant to show how the rape issue could be a metaphor, and by extension how "Annabel Chong" herself could be a Rorschach test, where people tend to interpret her according to their own presumptions and prejudices.

I know all about presumptions and prejudices because, like Annabel, I also left Singapore for similar reasons, in a quest for self-fulfillment through ways we both could never have dreamed of experiencing in our home country. And while I have myself made a long career out of reporting on various aspects of the sex industry, most prominently a ten-year cycle covering the adult film industry, Annabel Chong represented to me the darkest, deepest challenge of my professional life.

Succinctly put, could I suspend my own disbelief and apprehend her fairly, given that we were both of Chinese-Singaporean heritage and the fact that we both left the country largely for reasons of personal dissatisfaction with the status quo and we then both ended up working with adult entertainment?

Well, that was a Rorschach test I didn't need to take. It was obvious whose side of the fence I was on. Yet all the same, I was personally intrigued. For her, it wasn't enough to merely express angst-ridden rebellion by joining the uppermost ranks of the sex industry. She had to do something so ballsy, so far-out, and so out-there that she would surely capture your undivided attention.

That's what I needed to ponder, and what I needed to understand. And so I've written this book, based partly on my own relationship with her over the years (featuring, of particular note, three separate interviews done with her in the wake of the 1999 documentary), in an attempt to break new ground while exploring the numerous facets of the Annabel Chong legend: the mythological background of the gangbang genre (based on the Roman empress Messalina), the cult of the Asian pornstar (based on the "Asian fever" racial fetish), the phenomenon of social engineering in Singapore (based on our respective experiences), the arena of adult entertainment (both in the areas of film and video as well as the Internet) and, in its own glorious finality, the issue of celebrity and the mass-audience fixation with pop-culture outlaws like her.

Because hers was a celebrityhood with a difference. Porn is a form of commodified sex, packaged as a sizzling product for mass market consumption, and so she poses some fascinating questions: What does someone like Annabel Chong say about us, about the culture and society we live in? What is it that draws us to her mythology? "Annabel Chong is my hero," someone in Singapore once told me. "She dared to go there. I like to think she did it for us, so that we might challenge ourselves to go further in whatever we do in our lives."

Annabel herself went pretty far. In January 2002, *AVN* (*Adult Video News*, the official trade magazine of the American adult entertainment industry) published its list of the "Top 50 Pornstars of All Time," and the six stars at the top of the heap were Ron Jeremy, Jenna Jameson, John Holmes, Traci Lords, Linda Lovelace, and Marilyn Chambers. Annabel Chong came in at number 40, along with the following text:

The original mega-gangbang queen, Chong took on a purported 251 guys in The World's Biggest Gangbang – despite much disapproval from her fellow adult industry performers. She was quite intelligent and willing to perform in extreme-themed vids, doing anals and double penetrations with ease.

She made a number of movies, mainly for John T. Bone, before departing for parts unknown. She returned in the late '90s to help her director friend David Aaron Clark out by filling in at the last minute for a no-show performer.

The video was titled Poison Candy (Heatwave Entertainment) and may be her last sex role to date. She was also the subject of a mainstream documentary, Sex: The Annabel Chong Story.

"Poison candy" is what some people might consider pornography to be – the sexual equivalent of fast food, stuff that's tasty but which sometimes isn't all that good for you – yet a girl from Singapore placing in the Top 40 of porn's hallowed pantheon is, arguably, a remarkable achievement, despite how the aforesaid "disapproval from her fellow adult industry performers" was captured in a section from the documentary.

Several industry veterans were being interviewed at the annual *AVN* Expo, at the Sands convention center in Las Vegas, and they were seen commenting on the 1995 gangbang event in less than salutary ways.

"My first question is: Where did they get the guys?" the porn director Seymour Butts is seen asking. "Was there any health or safety in mind?"

"Let me ask you a question," the porn actress Ona Zee is seen asking. "How many times can you fuck 251 guys and still be okay? You can't. In your lifetime, what happens to you, internally, physically?

"It just gives porno a bad name," the porn actor Michael J. Coxx is seen saying. "When she did that, to me, it was like a slap in the face, to say porno is still really sleazy."

Even as recently as February 2011, the *LA Weekly* described the 1995 gangbang film as having "all the sex appeal of a *National Geographic* film of frogs spawning in a mud puddle." (She was described, with her real last name spelled wrong, as "Grace Kwek, a tiny Singaporean with the adopted stage name Annabel Chong.")

Regardless of such criticism, her being placed at number 40 on that *AVN* list isn't merely a benchmark for the record books. It also justifies my claim to a lofty ambition: that Annabel Chong as both myth and metaphor is worthy of due attention, and much can actually be learned from her fine if unconventional example.

1

PERSONA NON GRATIFICATION

There was once a time, back when the Internet was still in its infancy, when porn wasn't such a commonplace thing. When eyebrows were actually raised because a young woman from Singapore who called herself Annabel Chong came along and single-handedly (pardon the innuendo) changed the way we saw adult entertainment.

She broke new ground, because she did "reality" sex before the adjective was appended to television (and then to the newfound "tube site" craze spawned by *YouTube* and its more interesting adult cousin, *YouPorn*). People who know of her usually think of her solely in terms of that fateful day in January 1995, when she had sex 251 times in the course of ten hours. Not 251 men, as it has been claimed, but 251 "sex acts" – the polite euphemism for "penetrations." It was only revealed later that there were really only 70 men in attendance, who were "recycled" for extra rounds like guests at a buffet feast.

It was "reality" despite the dubious numbers, filmed for home video and made available to anyone who cared to see it. She didn't think it mattered, since she had meant it all to be a joke.

But, unfortunately, nobody got the point.

And the sheer irony of it all did not escape mention even on her *Wikipedia* page:

Chong sought to question the double standard that denies women the ability to exhibit the same sexuality as men, by modelling what a female "stud" would be. Skeptics suggest that, in reality, she merely brought art-school pretensions to a depiction of the culturally embedded "slut" stereotype. Other critics note that one can hold up historical gender biases for scrutiny without having sex with 70 men on camera.

The people in the adult film industry also missed the point, because they then started filming more gangbang events so that the last record could be broken. Jasmin St Claire did 300, Houston did 500, and on the eve of the big millennium, on New Year's Eve as the world counted out 1999, Sabrina Johnson supposedly did 2,000, over two days. It was a gimmick based on the number. And it backfired, too. (Sabrina later admitted she regretted doing it.)

Why spoil a spoof? The point of a gangbang was to poke fun at the number and question our assumptions about what sex really was about, anyway. By actually doing what it intended to warn us against, the American adult film producers were found wanting in the collective I.Q. department – a not uncommon situation in actuality, as all porn biz veterans will assure you.

You could say, however, that she was deserving of her fame because she was the very first one in the history books. It was like you forgot all the other guitar players once you heard Jimi Hendrix. (Well, Hendrix was quite the legendary Lothario, so it's an apt comparison.) Even in this modern age of media saturation, we can still be enthralled by the romance of provenance – nature abhors a vacuum and something must necessarily come from somewhere – even in these unctuous times when the shock value of hardcore porn has been severely compromised by the arrival of the Internet.

On September 16, 2009, Annabel herself discussed this with me by email, when she wrote: "The problem with the mainstreamization of porn is that now everybody is a pornstar – Kim Kardashian, those soldiers at Abu Ghraib, Verne Troyer. It makes performing sex for the camera common and banal. We have sites where couples are posting vids of themselves for free. Why pay for porn when everybody already has a sex tape to their name? Remember a decade ago when we had our first chat? I mentioned during that time that porn was the new rock & roll, since rock no longer has the power to shock – it has been co-opted into the mainstream. Well, I see the same thing happening to porn. It's no longer as taboo as it used to be. It's just what people do. And they do it all the time."

In my book about my years covering the American porn industry, *In Lust We Trust*, I recorded what Annabel had earlier told me: "Janine Lindemulder is the new Jimi Hendrix. And porn is the new rock & roll."

That was in 2005, five years before Janine Lindemulder found herself targeted by the tabloids during the sensational Hollywood divorce featuring actress Sandra Bullock and her bad-boy biker Jesse James. Lindemulder, James's ex-wife, was a former Vivid Video contract star who was (according to my own sources) still performing live webcam shows out of her own house to make ends meet after a six-month stint in prison for tax evasion; she had, as one gossip magazine alleged, set up his tryst with the tattooed stripper Michelle "Bombshell" McGee (who'd admitted in March 2010 that she had bedded James, catalyzing the marital split).

Once again, we folks in the porn trenches knew stuff, way before the civilians did. But, the "new rock & roll" notwithstanding, I myself wanted to return to what was really a more innocent time, if you can actually call it that. A time when you could even say that porn actually mattered. We're so jaded now that when pornstars make the news because of some scandalous event, we merely roll our eyes because it's just more banal news fodder. Like when the relatively unknown Capri Anderson (real name Christina Walsh) was reportedly paid US$12,000 by actor Charlie Sheen for just one night of fun at the Plaza Hotel in New York in October 2010. (Compare that to the US$10,000 Annabel Chong was offered for doing the 1995 gangbang, and ask yourself which deal was better?)

Or when it was disclosed in August 2005 that rugby star

Byron Kelleher of New Zealand's All Blacks national team was dating Asian-American pornstar Kaylani Lei ("Singapore-born sex kitten Ashley Spaulding a.k.a. Kaylani Lei, who has starred in 88 adult movies," as the *Asian Sex Gazette* website noted of her) or when pornstar Tanya Tate disclosed that Greg Jacob, a professional Irish hurler, had been one of her co-stars in her movie *Tanya Tate's Sex Tour of Ireland* ("I'm not ashamed of what I did," Jacob eventually admitted, after first denying it. "I just didn't want the family to know. It was just a bit of fun, it was a dare from the lads.")

And let's all spare a thought for Veronica Siwik-Daniels, a.k.a. pornstar Joslyn James, who had re-enacted her real-life affair with a certain golfer named Tiger Woods in her movie *The 11th Hole*, released by Vivid Entertainment under its Vivid-Celeb imprint in July 2010. Without Tiger, who would have heard of her outside the San Fernando Valley? He unintentionally gave her the kind of mainstream crossover appeal that she surely couldn't have even dreamed of. I mean, he even brought her to *my* attention; I myself hadn't heard of her before she made the news.

* * *

The host of the party, my friend Sonya Yeung, was telling a story to her guests at a barbeque dinner on Lamma Island in Hong Kong. She told them about a guy she knew who'd made a secondary career for himself by pilfering stuff from other people's websites and creating his own web portal out of them. He was rapidly aggregating colossal amounts of interesting information but was hosting this website from the server of the company he'd been working for.

One day, the company's webmasters noticed some highly unusual spikes in the server readings, all of which came not only from this particular guy's website but also from one predominant source: a film he had uploaded to his site, made in 1995 and called *The World's Biggest Gangbang,* starring a pornstar from Singapore named Annabel Chong. Quite likely, a lot of people had missed the boat back in 1995 and they were checking it out now.

But this was happening in 2008, a whole 13 years since the gangbang event that made her famous. I found it curious that there could still be so much ongoing interest in Annabel Chong after so much time had passed.

Perhaps there was currency in paradox, since her legend had been writ large because of her backstory – once a typical goody-two-shoes girl, a Chinese-Singaporean scholarship student to boot, then an unwilling target of tabloid frenzy simply because she had become the epicenter of a seismic shake-up in our ecology of sexual manners.

She had hid the truth from her own family, too; even her mother wouldn't know at all about her adult film career until she participated in the filming of the documentary *Sex: The Annabel Chong Story,* learning the truth as the cameras were rolling. Her mother is seen telling her only daughter to "regain my dignity" as the young woman weeps in shame.

The documentary was made in 1998, three whole years after the big gangbang itself, and its debut at the 1999 Sundance Film Festival led many a media pundit to speculate over its cultural worth.

Her real name, revealed as Grace Quek, alone invited clever wordplay. My own 1999 interview with her, which was how we first met, carried the headline "Grace Under Pressure" and what more fitting example of exhibiting grace under pressure could there be than being subjugated to the heaving, hirsute bodies of all those men?

Indeed, one of the very best things written about the whole phenomenon came from one of my favorite social commentators, Emily Jenkins, who noted in a piece (entitled "So Many Men") in *Mirabella* magazine, September 1999: "Most of us would find submitting to a 'gang bang' inherently degrading. But Quek sees it as a statement of erotic liberation. Still, she acknowledges that it is 'not exactly a PC idea of what a sexually enlightened female would do.'

"Funny and chatty, Quek slips easily from earnest feminist rhetoric to comical descriptions of her male co-stars' 'wood problems.' In that documentary, directed by Gough Lewis, she articulates the subversive view that her copulatory marathon actually satirizes masculinity while expressing the enormity of her own desire. To challenge our gender assumptions, Quek puts her body (and psyche) on the line, but the fact that the stunt was filmed for the pleasure of X-rated video enthusiasts and the profit of pornographers throws its political meaning into question.

"Lewis's documentary does not end happily. Quek devastates her mother with news of her career and revisits the site of a gang rape she survived years ago, which raises a troubling question: Is her adult-film work a way of punishing herself for that victimization, or of reclaiming her body?"

That final question is the best one ever asked about the motivations that lie behind lives devoted to sexual exhibitionism. Sex symbols exist more as conceptual entities rather than human personalities. Even in her native Singapore, people talk of Annabel Chong as if she were an urban myth.

And all because, I would argue, her very name only serves to beg a very loaded question: Who got there first, the celebrity or the slut?

Back in the 1990s, an American performance artist named Karen Finley often caught my attention, for reasons made obvious from this *Los Angeles Times* review by the theatre critic Laurie Stone: "Karen Finley often performs naked, and because she's gorgeous – long legs, round breasts, cascades of auburn hair, cheekbones out to here – nudity is a power position for her. She knows the audience approves of what she looks like. She can do whatever she wants with them."

And so, assuming we approve such power positions (even as we're also surely a tad envious), should engaging in sexually oriented performance be considered a serious career choice?

And should one deserve veneration or reproach if seen as a professional slut?

Some people might accept that kind of unconventional, fuck-you attitude with compassion and understanding, but I'd say they're usually worn with a blurry gauze of condescension – simply because of the ethical, moral and ultimately cultural slant occupied by the word "slut." A similar problem exists with the word "whore," one made worse by the Western cultural standard that defines pornography as "the writings of whores," now expanded in some quarters to include any visual depictions of women of questionable virtue.

My own view is that the tendency to censure or to judge based on such commonplace bias, often fuelled by religious rectitude, is what usually muddies the issue.

That's why the late Maria Schneider's performance in Bernardo Bertolucci's *Last Tango in Paris*, made in 1972, shocked so many people – the film received an "X" rating when it was first released in the United States, even with Marlon Brando in the cast, and it well and truly pushed the envelope. Bertolucci later explained that he came up with the movie's story line after he "dreamed of seeing a beautiful, nameless woman on the street and having sex with her without ever knowing who she was."

That line, right there, captured the very essence of what pornography is (or, more precisely, should be) about. Most scenes in porn movies certainly feature anonymous sex, the brazenly explicit version of Erica Jong's "zipless fuck" (as she put it in her 1973 novel *Fear of Flying*, another teenage touchstone for me), and it's precisely that kind of visual representation that we're addressing here.

However, more importantly, *Last Tango in Paris* was also my first exposure as a young teenager to what "pornography" was, even though I wouldn't actually see the film myself till many years later. It was banned in Singapore at the time but I found out about it from a report in *Time* magazine.

However, Maria Schneider (who died of cancer on February 3, 2011) was arguably upstaged that same year, 1972, by Linda Lovelace in *Deep Throat*, the film that dropped the phrase "porno chic" into the Western cultural lexicon. The anti-Nixon, post-hippie counterculture of the time certainly empowered it by supplying context, and it was almost certainly the first time most people in America had ever heard the term "pornstar" applied to anyone. I also thought it highly ironic that this bit of history had happened because of a movie about a woman whose clitoris lay in her throat, allowing her to orgasm from giving blowjobs, which put paid to the idea that vaginal sex was the only kind that qualified as real sex.

And then (still in 1972!), Marilyn Chambers came out of nowhere to indelibly imprint herself in many minds when she starred in a landmark porn film, *Behind The Green Door*, her fame enhanced by the revelation that she had also been the model emblazoned on boxes of *Ivory Snow* washing powder – to the embarrassment of its manufacturers Proctor & Gamble (who initially planned to remove her image from the boxes but relented after sales rose and they grudgingly gave Marilyn a five-year contract extension).

I still remember the first time I saw Marilyn Chambers – yes, she got there first, before I ever saw Linda Lovelace – so *Behind the Green Door* accrued far more cultural currency and Marilyn's star slung itself much higher for me in that particular exalted firmament (and hit a definite low when she died under sad and tragic circumstances in 2009, drunk and alone and living in a trailer). But she had already made her mark, paving the way for Paris Hilton. Gradually, the counterculture had been chipping away at the resistance of the more conservative factions, and things slowly started to give. After Jenna Jameson arrived with her bestselling book in 2001 and then Paris Hilton arrived with her home video in 2004, the walls truly came tumbling down.

In retrospect, we see the delightfully tacky *One Night in Paris* as a landmark event in pop culture history – the first time a homemade porn video had actually boosted rather than jeopardized someone's fledgling career, even making Paris Hilton a household name. Pamela Anderson's own sex tape scandal had made news some years earlier but this was different – Pamela Anderson was then already an established star, whereas many people only came to know of Paris Hilton *because* of this supposedly scandalous event.

Was it rigged to generate publicity for her? We may never know. But what I do know is this – a whole 15 years ago, back in 1995, that would never have happened.

Back in 1995, when Annabel Chong took cultural rebellion to an extreme, on terms that had never been negotiated before. And history was really being made, even while many of its participants were completely clueless about its eventual significance.

And that, I think, remains her most lasting cultural value.

*   *   *

People do strange things to spite the societies they come from. I can personally attest to the profundity of this, having covered the adult film business myself for an equally long stretch of time.

I'd started, coincidentally, in the spring of 1995 when I began working for the *Spice* adult-cable television company, just as news of the then-biggest gangbang was fresh on the airwaves. I had seen for myself how the psychological make-up of so many of these young women constituted a double-edged sword. I learned that exposing yourself as completely as possible was also a way of taking back what had been taken from you – innocence, trust, and youth – because, however they often hated to admit it, most of the girls really had their careers founded in events from childhood, usually either a by-product of childhood abuse or of abandonment and neglect, or (worse) a combination of all of the above.

Whatever Annabel's were, however, I don't quite know. She never told me because I never asked.

I almost never brought up the subject with any sex worker I dealt with, unless they themselves volunteered it, because it's a highly invasive question that often only elicits defensive posturing or outright lies. Anyone can understand that – nobody wants to admit to a total stranger they've just met, let alone a reporter, that they were sexually abused as a child.

I only know she had issues with her father but they patched things up shortly before he died, and that she remains close to her mother. The nearest I ever got to any answer of that nature was when we were discussing our shared issues with the way we had both grown up amid the squeaky-clean, uptight environment that had tellingly defined Singapore for too many years.

In the first interview we did together, in 1999, she echoed a statement she had also made in the documentary film. She told me: "I don't think Singapore is for everybody. There are people who take well to the system and thrive on it. And, well, good for them. But for me, personally, I don't think that it is a system that sits well with me politically."

I then said to her, as recorded in our interview: "One of the problems I find with Singapore society is that people are spoon-fed short cuts to success, to make them feel the government has the answers."

She agreed: "The way the government posits itself as a father, like 'father knows best.' A lot of people swallow that idea … It's very insidious … And I guess living in Los Angeles gives me enough space to resist it."

That last statement resonated with me, since I had also left the country for similar reasons. When I arrived in Los Angeles in 1984, I instantly felt like I was home. The first few times I went to see bands in the rock clubs of West Hollywood, I was struck by the realization that there were people like me – social misfits to a degree, all sharing a subcultural identity.

To deal with the mythology of Annabel Chong is to deal with those kinds of issues. And being "progressive" in Singapore, if you ask those very people, means challenging the system in numerous subtle ways. Even though Annabel Chong, as their *de facto* patron saint, was hardly subtle in her methodology.

Yet she is that very rebellion incarnate. Annabel Chong doing *The World's Biggest Gangbang* was like a comet blazing across the skies with shock 'n' awe splendor, driving the natives out of the woods to gasp and gawk.

* * *

People often ask me the same old question: "What is Annabel Chong like as a real person?"

My immediate thought, which I don't usually say aloud, is: "What is anyone like as a real person? Can anyone really know?"

That question is always a loaded one. Most people have no direct access to women they've only heard or read about (or seen on video, in the case of their favorite pornstars), so they're always interested to know if whatever I say matches the preconceived notions in their heads. While Grace Quek, her real name, has been widely strewn in places both in print and online hither and yon, much less ink has been devoted to Annabel Chong as a mythological sex goddess and take-all-comers gangbang queen.

There are, for instance, hardly any compelling analyses of the by-products of her mythology – what sociologists call the "parasocial" nature of celebrity worship, a one-way-traffic phenomenon where attention is fixated on an individual who herself has little or no interest in her own audience.

I know this phenomenon quite well, because I had been everybody's go-to person since 1999. All kinds of people wrote to me, asking me to forward requests to interview her, usually from the media. One magazine editor asked me to contact her about a project he was assembling about "famous girls" from her alma mater, Raffles Girls' School. A television reporter wanted to talk to her for his show about sexual health and HIV/AIDS. There was even a request from academia – from one Melissa Garcia Knoll, a doctoral candidate at the University of California, Riverside, seeking an interview with Annabel Chong for her dissertation about "how women of color deploy sexuality and the erotic to open up new avenues for empowerment." (Yes, in the United States, Asian women were still considered "women of color" despite the obvious racial-profiling implications.)

Most of the time, I declined all requests on her behalf.

Only one was granted by Annabel – Melissa Garcia Knoll, because she was asking sincerely as an academic and not as a nosy reporter. It became glaringly obvious to me what Annabel thought of the press.

However, she never once turned me down whenever I asked for an interview, no matter how complex or simple. For instance, for the February 2001 issue of *Penthouse Variations*, I wrote a long piece called "Pornstar Rock" about pornstars who were involved with rock music, and it included a sidebar in which I asked several pornstars one deceptively simple question: "What do you like to listen to when you're having sex?" Some of the answers were somewhat predictable (names like Enya, Sade, Kiss, and Pink Floyd came up) and two of them (Asia Carrera and Janine Lindemulder) said "nothing" because music "would kill the mood." Annabel, on the other hand, immediately answered: "Underground club music, anything that's drum and bass. I don't have any favorite artists - it's not about the artist, it's more about just the music. It's about setting a mood that's great for sex."

The girl was a real slave to rhythm. In such light, I myself was sympathetic to Annabel's own glee at subverting the stereotype of the shy, submissive Asian girl. Going the whole hog and getting yourself filmed gangbanging a bunch of guys, now wasn't that sexually liberating?

Yet where was that fine line, between empowerment and enslavement?

On a personal level, I had always been intrigued by the

concept of "consensual degradation" in porn. I'll never forget Sasha Grey's stunning debut performance in John Stagliano's 2006 film *Fashionistas Safado: The Challenge* (the second part of his *Fashionistas* trilogy) – I can still remember my own amazement when I learned after the fact that it was her first-ever porn movie at the age of 18, and she'd *chosen* an orgy scene to mark the occasion, too! A petite little girl being pounded by guys twice her size – I lost count because of the fast cuts in editing but I think she fucked at least five of them – and because it was her first movie, she was ripe and ready and matched every one of them stroke for stroke. It's still one of the all-time standout scenes in American porn.

At the 2007 *AVN* Awards, she shared the "Best Group Sex Scene" trophy with the other performers in that scene and she herself won the big one, "Female Performer of the Year" – a rarity, for a new girl to win that in her very first year in the business, but she certainly deserved it. (And it led to bigger things, like being cast the following year as the lead actress in Steven Soderbergh's film *The Girlfriend Experience*, in which she played a US$2,000-an-hour Manhattan escort.)

However, appearing onscreen having sex and then being recognized for what you did, those were the very things some of these girls didn't always care to discuss. Within the industry itself, it was easy enough – I had no trouble with any of the women I met and profiled ever opening up to me when I was writing about them for *Penthouse Variations* or *AVN Online*, but being subjected to the coarse attention of mainstream newspapers and magazines, that was something else. You were dealing with whole audiences who weren't already converted, who had to be persuaded that you weren't mentally ill or borderline psychotic.

For instance, witness the most laughable example of *fait accompli* support, in the form of Singapore's very amusing tabloid, *The New Paper*, which noted on August 19, 2008 that Annabel Chong had outgrown the industry that made her famous and was now a devoted marathon runner when she wasn't working her day job as a web developer in Los Angeles. "*Annabel is Dead: From Sex Marathons to Real Marathons*" sang the headline, and the piece noted that "she's also into golf, yoga, pilates, dancing, hiking, organic food, and is a self-proclaimed 'sports nut' and is a huge fan of several baseball and American football teams." It was almost as if the litany of sporting interests was needed to justify her newfound life (the none-too-subtle subtext being "sports is better than porn").

I did blanch slightly when I read my own name in the same story – local theatre director Loretta Chen finally "managed to contact her through Mr Gerrie Lim, author of *Invisible Trade: High-Class Sex for Sale in Singapore*, and a personal friend of Ms Quek's" – but what I found most telling was the way the piece ended, with this curious coda:

The New Paper was the first in Singapore to break Annabel Chong's story on 27 Jan 1997.

The article, Annabel's chosen profession and her record-breaking sexual feat shocked and scandalised many.

But there were also those who couldn't help but marvel – morality aside – at the Singaporean who dared to do the unthinkable, the elitely-educated middle-class girl who, ironically, fulfilled the very Singaporean obsession about breaking world records and putting Singapore on the world map.

What a contrite tone of voice, I thought, almost diametrically opposite that previously adopted by the same paper. In 1999, it ran a piece on the documentary's premiere at the Cannes Film Festival with the headline "Amazing Dis-Grace."

"She's trying to fit as many as possible into her tight schedule," observed the reporter blithely, of her Cannes publicity schedule, adding that those who did score interviews "can now truthfully say they had a short-time Annabel Chong … I would have called her 'Amazing Grace' but that would have soiled, smeared and sullied a truly beautiful song."

The paper's bragging rights – of how it first broke the story in Singapore on January 27, 1997 – made no mention of the obvious irony: This was almost *two* years to the day after the record-setting gangbang of January 19, 1995.

And so, in karmic retribution, the universe decreed that Singapore's only contribution to global popular culture would be a pornstar named Annabel Chong. Which made perfect sense to me.

* * *

My first actual contact with Annabel was in 1999, when I interviewed her after being introduced by producer David Whitten, a connection made possible by then-programmer Philip Cheah of the Singapore International Film Festival.

She said to me: "You have to understand that Annabel Chong is a persona, she's a character. I think the dichotomy is interesting. I think everybody puts on personas, although their personas may not necessarily have a different name."

That's true of all celebrities, of course, and you have to understand a person's chosen persona to fully appreciate its intended guise. As the '70s shock-rock icon Alice Cooper once noted in an *Esquire* magazine interview, the way to become a living legend is to create a legendary character and then "leave that character on the stage." In this manner, a celebrity lets his or her fans project their fantasies onto that stage character, that persona, while he or she goes on with the usual process of dealing with regular life. (I'd once interviewed Cooper myself, and he gleefully confirmed this to be the very secret of his longevity.)

However, there was a fundamental problem when this was applied to porn, itself being a subcultural genre of pop culture that only the most perverse of sensibilities (like mine) can fully appreciate.

Take, for example, Larry Flynt's clever mantra for his Hustler Hollywood stores, "Relax, it's just sex!" For a lot of people, I'm willing to wager, sex happens to be the very one thing they'd be least relaxed about.

In one of the best interviews that emerged from the *Sex: The Annabel Chong Story* media circus of 1999, fellow Asian-American writer Rosy Ngo, in the September/October 1999 issue of *Pop Smear* magazine, asked her: "Were you bored during the gang bang?"

"There were points when I was frustrated," Annabel replied, "because I vibe into people – when people are nervous, I get twice as nervous, and some of the guys got very nervous. I don't blame them because it's their first time in front of a camera and they have to be able to perform in front of all the lights, in front of all these other men. It's just difficult. And if they fail, guess what? They fail on video – more pressure! So they're really nervous, and they've gotten me really nervous and frustrated. It's like, 'Come on, relax!' It's only a video, dammit!"

And there's the whole problem, right there. As all good pornstars have been wont to know (and naive newbies are often shocked to discover), appearing naked and performing in front of fully rolling cameras is an act that lasts *forever*. You can download anything off the Internet these days.

As veteran porn actress Jill Kelly once told me, there were girls she knew who were dismayed over their limited career options. "A lot of girls need to realize you can't leave and try to get a job at Nordstrom's or at a shopping mall," she said. "They might get fired because somebody found out they're a pornstar."

My own real interest, however, always lay with how the

actual persona that had been created actually outlasted the actual career that made it necessary.

Look up "Annabel" on *Wikipedia* and you'll see that it's "a female given name, a variant of Amabel probably influenced by Anna," which arose in Scotland during the Middle Ages though its main usage has been in English and Dutch. And "Annabel Chong (a.k.a Grace Quek (pornographic actress)" occupies fifth place in *Wikipedia*'s list of famous usages of the name (following the 1906 novel *Annabel* by L. Frank Baum, a song performed by Maria Dimitriadi, the British actress Annabelle Apsion and the English socialite Annabel Astor).

My own introduction to the name was by way of the last poem written by Edgar Allan Poe that I had read when I was an impressionable teenager, "Annabel Lee." Would "Annabel Lee" have been too obvious an *homage*, even though it sounds like a great name for an Asian pornstar?

Interestingly, as I write, there is now an American pornstar named Annabelle Lee, who is not Asian but is "white as white can be, and, for the record, is also a fan of Poe," to quote director Melissa Monet, who had shot Annabelle in her all-girl film *Blu Dreams 2*, released in October 2010. (I have no idea why she altered the spelling – perhaps she feared litigation from the Poe estate.)

Would Poe have turned in his grave? On the contrary, methinks, from my own reading of his books, that he would probably have approved. No flattery quite like imitation, and all that jazz.

Pornstardom has now become part of modern popular culture, thanks to certain names that loom large in this context: Tera Patrick, the reigning Asian-American porn queen (and her own memoirs, cheekily entitled *Sinner Takes All*); Julianne Moore and Heather Graham as pornstars in *Boogie Nights*; Heather Graham as the reluctant pornstar in Daisy von Scherler Mayer's 2002 Bollywood spoof *The Guru*; and the brilliant yet under-appreciated Juliette Marquis in my own favorite mainstream film about a fictitious pornstar, *This Girl's Life* (released in 2003 with the catchy ad slogan: "When love is your business, what do you do for pleasure?"). Lindsey Lohan, of course, almost made the list until November 2010, when they rescinded her latest job, the lead role in the Linda Lovelace biopic *Inferno*, thanks to her serial drug-rehab habit.

Some might claim the closest thing to Annabel Chong was Felicia Tang, the *Playboy TV* model and softcore starlet, but the similarities really ended at the birthplace – Felicia Tang was indeed born in Singapore but grew up in Perth, Western Australia, before moving to Los Angeles where she built a potentially successful career that included minor roles in some mainstream movies (she appeared in *Cradle 2 The Grave*, *Rush Hour 2*, and *The Fast and The Furious*), though this ascent was abruptly halted in September 2009 (when, at age 31, she was brutally murdered by her boyfriend, a former church pastor).

A more fitting spiritual sister to Annabel was someone Felicia Tang had worked with – in 2003, she had appeared in an erotic online video with another Singapore-born celebrity, the vivacious Tila Tequila, in which both women appeared nude and fondled each other in a swimming pool. Tequila, the hip-hop star and MTV television host, was born Tila Nguyen in Singapore of Vietnamese parents who'd fled their war-torn homeland, but she then grew up in Houston, Texas. The young Tila, at age 18, was discovered by a *Playboy* talent scout at a shopping mall and she did a nude centerfold test shoot, eventually becoming the *Playboy* website's first-ever Asian "Cyber Girl of the Month."

Her notoriety later spread through several strategic career moves – she admitted in the April 2006 issue of *Stuff* magazine that she adopted her stage name from her love of alcohol (she'd started drinking when she was 13), and in April 2010 she released a song through iTunes entitled "I Fucked the DJ." She also got into a public scuffle in August 2010 with a group of Juggalos (fans of the rock band Insane Clown Posse) at a concert in Illinois; she claimed the men had pelted her with rocks and faeces but a witness reported this happening only after she had taunted them and taken her top off, allegedly inciting them to violence.

That, to me, was an example of true celebrity branding, however berserk and bizarre. Tila Tequila actually deployed her sexuality to her advantage without actually being a *bona fide* pornstar, arguably achieving more by doing less. This might well be so if you consider double- and triple-penetration scenes a lot more hard work (so to speak), let alone multiple gangbangs.

Annabel Chong had done all those – she was credited as the groundbreaking recipient in American porn's very first triple-penetration scene, taking a penis in her vagina and two in her anus in the film *Depraved Fantasies #3* – but *Wikipedia* singles out only five of her 52 official films for particular mention:

Annabel started in porn by answering an advertisement in the LA Weekly, which led to photo shoots and then an interview with director John T. Bone. Bone, recognizing Chong's talent, embarked on producing a series of films starring her. She was the new hardcore princess in "Sgt. Pecker's Lonely Hearts Club Gangbang" and "I Can't Believe I Did The Whole Team." In "Anal Queen" and "Depraved Fantasies #3," Annabel took hardcore pornography to a new level when she pioneered on-camera triple penetration.

The production that propelled Annabel into the limelight was another John T. Bone production, "The World Biggest Gang Bang." Chong advertised on adult television for 300 participants for the event. Even though only seventy or so participants showed up, this still caused a sensation in the porn world. As well as being the single largest grouping of men ever, Annabel had started a new trend. There were even more gangbangs, but none were as famous.

Five notable films out of an official 52 – what does that tell us? That the other films were disposable and forgettable?

They forgot her directorial debut *Pornomancer*, in which she starred alongside "gonzo" goddess Alana Evans, and they also forgot *I Love Asians #5* ("Don Fernando has an Oriental itch … and super cock sucker Annabel Chong offers him some fabulous fortune cookie nookie!"), *More Dirty Debutantes #37* (her first porn appearance at the grubby horndog hands of the infamous Ed Powers, who was besotted by her "British accent") and the oh-so-cute *Straight A's* (she appears on the box cover clad in a graduation cap and gown, topless and wearing just a thong, inspiring apt promotional copy – "Professor of Filth, John T. Bone says with a smile: 'Annabel is great, I wish I had a hundred students like her. Annabel Chong is at the top of her class! She is a fantastic student who enjoys "cramming" and tutoring new freshmen who have hard subjects!'")

Were these films denied recognition because the sex seemed repetitive? But why should that be such a bad thing? Porn, after all, derives its power from repetition – because masturbation depends greatly on the hypnotic pleasure of repetitive motion, much like the transcendence of a three-chord blues progression. (Well, almost.)

No, you might dislike the message but don't shoot the messenger. Pornstars are really brave pawns in a larger chess game, performers serving a director's manifesto.

They are, ultimately, representations of sexual energy, manifest through the medium of video technology, a justifiable expression of democratic principles built upon freedom of expression. Neither you nor I should condemn it just because we personally don't get turned on by what we see, be they big-titted midgets or bingo-winged fatsos or raisin-shrivelled grannies – or what-have-you, even as we all rightfully choose to draw the line at underaged children and farm animals.

*   *   *

And that, as they say, was where Annabel Chong came in.

And her example is particularly noteworthy. Because she'd grown up, like me, in a young country whose government founded its principles on self-proclaimed Confucian paternalism, manifested in an obsession with social engineering. But all that really did was drive forward those lovable forces of Newtonian physics: For every action, there is an equal and opposite reaction. Create a nanny state so that people will stay "obedient" and you've simultaneously created a backlash, via a sector of the population who will attempt to free themselves of their metaphysical shackles.

I know this to be true because, like Annabel, I was one of them. Annabel Chong did it by creating a persona to service her rebellion, an alter-ego more profoundly powerful than the real person.

And when that persona is a sexually themed one, with all the implicit charm of a loaded gun, it becomes a larger-than-life transformation and the very pinnacle of celebrity-branding success, achieving what modern brand marketers like to call "singularity" – that very quality that makes an individual so highly prized that they are co-opted into the mechanism of branding. Marketing buzzwords can be highly deceptive, but "singularity" usually occurs when someone possesses a set of uniquely attractive characteristics.

So what made Annabel Chong attractive when she established the very "singularity" of her brand?

It was hardly the porn *per se*, if you ask me; Jenna Jameson's *My Plaything*, produced in November 2000, was a lot more revolutionary since it was filmed to service the cause of surrogate sex, with Jenna sighing and writhing in all kinds of positions shot from the viewer's P.O.V. ("It's totally interactive so it's like you're having sex with me," Jenna brightly declared, when I met and interviewed her in 2001. "I know that if I was a guy, it would be the ultimate jack-off – every man who watches this is going to want to fuck me!")

Back in January 1995, however, that kind of virtual reality wasn't so readily available, simply because the P.O.V. camera technology just wasn't there yet. So Annabel did it her way, using what she had back then. She utilized the vehicle of the multiple-man gangbang.

There was a parallel to Jenna Jameson's *My Plaything*, of course – the aim was to make every guy watching *want* to have sex with Annabel Chong, despite the inferior quality of the final execution. Its relatively cheap-and-cheerful, "gonzo"-style production values were hardly the point, anyway. Shock value was the currency being traded.

Some people got it. (And, of course, some didn't. Like anything in the wacky world of pop culture.) Famous American novelists like Chuck Palahniuk and Bret Easton Ellis wrote about her, revealing diametrically opposite reactions to the Annabel Chong phenomenon.

Palahniuk devoted several pages to her in his droll 2008 porn-parody novel *Snuff*, writing in a jaunty vernacular that underscored the sense of farce:

Miss Chong's best skill was crowd management. It was her idea to bring the men into the set in groups of five. Among those five, the first man got erect was the one got to screw her. Each group was on set ten minutes, and whoever was able got to ejaculate. Even if some guys never got hard, never touched her, all five counted towards the 251-man total.

The real genius was to make it a competition. The erection race.

Ellis, on the other hand, wrote what might well be the nastiest review of *Sex: The Annabel Chong Story*, in the July/ August 1999 issue of the now defunct *Gear* magazine. He noted (following the ominous headline: "She's Faking It – You Can Tell: The Annabel Chong Story Sucks") that "Grace Quek may be a decent student who knows how to write anthropology papers but when trying to verbalize her motivations within the context of being a pornstar she comes off as a babbling idiot."

"Grace Quek is a naughty provocateur but she's also an airhead, who actually seems more knowing and direct when playing bimbo cheerleaders in porn films," he concluded. "She's just an extreme individual whose behavior got her a lot of publicity. She's also a put-on artist who comes off as a phony." But he nearly nailed it, though, when he wrote that "instead of seeing a young woman standing up for sexual liberation through self-abasement, what you're really watching is a portrait of screwed-up post-adolescent rebellion based on the conservatism of an upbringing."

Naturally, the real Annabel hated Ellis for that review ("That Bret Easton Ellis," she told me, "his new novel sucks pigeon shit!") though I actually thought Ellis partially correct for that one observation, albeit too simplistically put.

But I also thought it curious that Ellis could denigrate "screwed-up post-adolescent rebellion" when he himself deployed the very same thing as both theme and subject of his own bestselling novels, notably the first three (*Less Than Zero*, *The Rules of Attraction* and *American Psycho*).

Perhaps it took a one-trick pony to know another?

2

MESSALINA'S REVENGE

They said she needed an ice pack, so she could ice down her swollen pussy. And some of the men were admonished by director John "T. Bone" Bowen on his megaphone, for digging their fingernails into her inner thighs.

Apocrypha or maledicta? Truth or rumor? (Or, more to the point, truth or dare?) Didn't it make for better publicity anyway, in the end? One of my favorite Bob Dylan songs, "Silvio," comes to mind: "Every pleasure's got an edge of pain, so pay for your ticket and don't complain."

The very idea of being gangbanged might be the apex of "consensual degradation" in porn, but it's actually not the act itself that interests me; I have always been far more intrigued with the bigger picture, the larger issue – that of our sexual boundaries, and why we all differ in our respective sexual comfort levels.

"I need to see my audience," the stripper I'd once dated declared to me, explaining why she could never do porn. "I don't mind spreading my legs and showing pink on stage, but the idea of an anonymous audience – guys out there at home watching me in their living rooms, jacking off and jizzing away – *that* just creeps me out!"

Well, try telling that to a pornstar who does gangbangs.

She'd probably say *not* being filmed while you're putting out your pussy, that's just stupidity. To quote once more one of my favorite people in porn, Jill Kelly, who told me: "I once worked at a club called Peepshow, where the guys jack-off and you're standing there, behind glass. I know girls who will do gangbangs but they won't do that. It just blows me away."

At any rate, for most pornstars who agree to be seen servicing any number of guys, there's only one thing to keep in mind, best articulated by the French pornstar Rebecca Lord. When I interviewed her in October 1999, we discussed her movie *Gangbang Girl #14*, and she told me: "I like doing them. I do. If I had to find one criticism of it, I would say this – when I have sex with a partner, I really like to take care of him, and in a gangbang you get so many guys around you, you can't take care of them. You have to let them take care of you. So it's nice, but it's different."

Was Annabel Chong thinking this on that day in January 1995? Nobody really knows except her own good self, though I would bet my last dollar that it wasn't as nice as it could've been. When gangbangs are shot in the pristine serenity of a movie soundstage, the mood is quite different – more concentrated and almost solemn, akin to a religious ritual – whereas the sheer spectacle of her much more public event must have lent an unexpectedly surreal edge to the proceedings.

There was just no way those guys, going at it five at a time, would "take care" of her in the way Rebecca had meant. Instead of a harmonious group therapy session of sorts, what we saw on video was a woman giving herself up like a piece of meat in the basest, bestial way.

And in a perverse sense, that was apropos – because the gangbang was really just an excuse for a larger, more profound agenda. I believe she was motivated by things that went beyond just expecting some studs to "take care of her" – she was much more ambitious than that. That would explain why she cited the example of Valeria Messalina, the promiscuous Roman empress, as the inspiration for her own sexual vision quest.

"John Bowen, the owner of the company who used to direct my videos, I basically challenged him to come up with a crazy idea for me to do," she told writer Amy Goodman in an interview with *Nerve*, the literary erotica journal, "and he came up with *The World's Biggest Gangbang*. I thought it was very amusing. When he first told me, I just laughed.

"And I thought about it for a while and I'm like, you know, 'Hey, let's do it.' During that time a friend of mine coincidentally mentioned something to me about the Roman empress Messalina, who apparently invited the entire town of Rome to have sex with her. It was a challenge to the top prostitute of Rome, and Messalina apparently won. So, I kind

49

of had that idea in mind, and that's why the entire video had this bizarre Roman theme that looked really cheesy."

Yes, all those Roman columns and gurgling fountains seen in the movie were attempts to replicate a historical backdrop. Annabel Chong served up herself as postmodern homage to Valeria Messalina.

*　*　*

Here's the history lesson, the short version of the long story.

The Roman empress Messalina (sometimes spelled Messallina) was the third wife of the emperor Claudius and also the paternal cousin of Nero, the second cousin of Caligula and the great-grandniece of Augustus. She was born in AD 20 and died in AD 48 – dying at age 28 at the sword of an assassin hired by Claudius himself, after he'd learned that Messalina had earlier attempted to have him murdered so that her new lover, the Roman senator Gaius Silius, could usurp the throne. (Claudius was at a dinner when she was killed; when the news was brought to him, he showed no emotion and merely asked for more wine.)

There are some minor discrepancies in the historical record – Messalina, at age 18, was supposedly forced as a practical joke by Caligula to marry Claudius, a dimwit 30 years older than her, though others theorize that Claudius, being Caligula's paternal uncle, married her to strengthen his own ties to the imperial family. Whatever the case, they both ascended to the throne in AD 41 when Caligula was murdered and Messalina became the most powerful woman in the Roman empire. Claudius had statues of her erected in various public places and her birthday officially celebrated.

Rather pointedly, she was accorded the privilege of front seats at the theatre alongside the Vestal Virgins – virgins consecrated to the goddess Vesta whose job was to tend to her temple's ever-burning sacred fire.

But, of course, no virgin was Messalina herself (and did she have an ever-burning fire, between her legs). Two historians have noted her rapacious sexual appetite for both senators and slaves, and she even worked at a brothel under an assumed name (or, as one other version had it, had owned a brothel and organized orgies for Roman women of the upper classes). Still, her biggest claim to fame, as recorded by the historian Pliny the Elder in Book X of his *Natural History*, lay in one historic occasion – when she challenged the most famous prostitute of Rome to a fucking contest, to see who could have sex with more men in a single night.

The prostitute was apparently named Scylla – not named by Pliny but by two others (the Restoratian playwright Nathaniel Richards in his 1640 play *The Tragedy of Messalina, Empress of Rome* and the novelist Robert Graves in his book *Claudius the God*) – and the contest was won by Messalina, when Scylla gave up after her twenty-fifth stud.

That was the none-too-subtle subtext of *The World's Biggest Gangbang* circa January 1995, hence the faux-Roman set with the toga-attired cast and crew. Messalina's record was broken, Annabel herself once said in interviews, in the 1980s by "a madam working in Amsterdam, who took 125 men. But, to my knowledge, that event was not captured on video."

Aha, therein lay the difference! Messalina and Scylla had to rely on the local scribes of the day, so we have no visual record of that contest either! One would have thought John Bowen should've been anointed a Badass Genius of the Year award of some sort for his foresight.

But in retrospect, what he really did was use the camera to record sex as spectacle and unknowingly usher in the age of reality-based "gonzo" porn a few years before the genre itself took hold of the American consciousness. Somewhere between 1999 and 2000, gonzo became the porn of choice for most consumers and this irrevocably changed the adult entertainment marketplace.

And when the gangbang meets the gonzo in a merger of sub-genres, the limitations of "reality" are well and truly stretched – because gangbanging is an extreme case of sexual representation. A pornstar's job, conventionally, is to project sexual availability, even though she might not actually be available, but when a girl does a gangbang she is arguably projecting the very opposite: She is supposedly implying that she is very much available indeed. Any guy, it seems, will do.

The big gangbang of 1995 was actually the end of an era, even though none of its participants knew it at the time.

* * *

In the aforesaid *Nerve* interview, Annabel was asked about the mechanics of performing that day, and she noted that not everyone wore condoms. Some of her studs were "professionals" who had been regularly tested, so they were excluded from the condom-only policy for the regular guys. "They took them off when coming, but they didn't come inside me," she disclosed. "The thing about porn is that they want everything to be visible so the internal cumshot is just sort of pointless. It's this really bizarre idea of sex, where it's not sex for the purpose of pleasure but sex for the purpose of visibility."

That visibility was also certified in two other ways that day.

Firstly, all the men had to be naked while waiting in line. "They were all naked because we wanted to prevent them from carrying concealed weapons. I wanted to prevent the situation of having an anti-porn guy who thinks this is really depraved coming out with a pistol and, like, blowing my brains out.

"Yeah, that wouldn't be good."

And secondly, they fudged the numbers to make it appear like they would make their original target of 250 studs (with Ron Jeremy designated number 251 by John Bowen himself at the end, as a digestif following a fully sated meal). This is what most people don't know, or didn't get the chance to know, because of the publicity circus around the event itself.

In that same *Nerve* interview, Annabel herself came clean:

The plan was five at a time for ten minutes, but what eventually happened was that if the guys were good and strong, they'd let them go on for longer than ten minutes. If the guys were kind of limp and they weren't able to get into it, they'd move them on ... They didn't have to penetrate me. It's just five guys on the stage and when they go off the stage, it counts as five ... Most of it would be them taking turns trying to get hard and the first person who gets hard would have sex with me and then I would see another guy getting hard and I'd point to him and say, "Your turn now." And I was really surprised that the guys were really polite about taking turns; they didn't fight on stage, things did not get unpleasant or pushy. That was one of my main concerns, that a fight would break out and things would get ugly.

Now, wasn't that a spectacle to end all spectacles? Guys waiting in line, stud-horses jammed in a paddock, ushered in groups of five, only ten minutes per group. Orgasms were not the point at all, since they had to finish in ten minutes whatever the status. And the cumshots that were shot were done specifically for the requisite camera angles since it *was* porn, after all, and those jetting sperm blasts were simply *de rigeur*, designed to fit the archetypal male notion of sexual "completion."

Annabel herself estimates that only about 30 percent of the men actually "finished":

We recycled the guys, actually, because some of them – the first time they went out they didn't manage to do it because they were nervous, and maybe they managed to do it the second time … Yeah. Everybody got to go.

And that, boys and girls, is all you really needed to know about that fateful day, at least in terms of the elements that mattered.

All the rest is, permit the unfortunate expression, fluff. (There were indeed some fluffer girls in attendance, planted to service not only the men but the age-old myth that "fluffers" exist on porn sets, to prepare male talent with either handjobs or blowjobs – in reality, however, they don't exist at all; in 15 years, I myself have never seen a fluffer on any porn set.)

The film itself is very much faux-documentary – a lot of boring preparatory psychobabble preceding the gangbang itself, interviews with the key participants, Bowen briefing Annabel and the guys, a press interview with Annabel, Annabel re-emerging in a gown and finally climbing onto the stage bed. She then grins and sassily reclines in readiness, as Bowen calls out for the first five participants.

*　*　*

It's probably worth nothing that the British-born Bowen previously served time as male porn talent himself, working under the name Harry Horndog, though he's still really only best known for having directed those two gangbang epics (*The World's Biggest Gangbang 2*, starring Jasmin St Claire, was released in 1996) – that's just two out of his 300-plus movies, made for several American porn studios (most notably Metro, VCA, New Sensations and Zane Entertainment).

In 1997, he tried to reinvent himself with a new company, Cream Entertainment, which proved disastrous, shutting down in 2000. He then moved to Brazil, where he operated a porn studio in Sao Paolo in 2004, making movies with the Brazilian soap opera star Alexandra Frota. He made the news again in April 2007 when he was arrested in Pattaya, Thailand, for allegedly shooting porn in an apartment he'd rented. Two of his associates were also arrested (Kyle Micgram, known in America as Vin Cross of Hustler's *Asian Fever* fame, and Thai-American talent scout Paul Sangsuwan a.k.a Chuk Wow, the transexual porn director of such titles as *Ladyboys in Latex*).

Pornography production is illegal in Thailand, punishable with jail terms of up to three years, and on April 6, 2007 the *Pattaya Daily News* reported:

On entering the apartment, they found pornography and video equipment for making porn and all kinds of sex equipments, as well as VCDs and photos ... The police, upon further exploration of another two rooms, found one room had been decorated as a large, fully-equipped studio with lights, flash equipment and a big video camera for taking movies and photos. They also found sexy dresses, black leather hot pants, etc., to clothe their actors and actresses.

Significantly, the porno filmmakers had placed Buddha images in the corner of every room to make sure that every photo or video they took would show the Buddha images in them. They also made the actresses dress up in Thai costumes which they made them take off, piece by piece, while taking the video.

The police, on checking some video movies, found the filmmakers were using katueys dressed up as woman ... These had starred in some very raunchy, sadistic and wild movies, which had been then uploaded to the Internet ...

Mr John Gilbert Bowen admitted he had rented the apartment in question some five months ago and confessed that he had set it up as a large, sophisticated studio to make X-rated movies and also to set up a website, mainly to run it as a large business with his friend. He had hired Mr Kyle Mark Micgram, who is also his closest friend and a specialist in photography, to operate the business together ... They had then hired bar girls or katueys to act in the movies ... Mr Paul, who is Thai-American and speaks fluent English, is in charge of looking for girls to star in the movie and to be the interpreter during the operation.

Mr John Gilbert Bowen said his was not the only website that is dedicated to the porn business; there are literally thousands of them. As most of the customers of these porn sites are foreigners, Bowen considered they should not be illegal. If the police want to arrest him, he continued, then they should arrest those who run every other porn website, as well.

However, the police were not of the same opinion, and informed the porn makers that their practice is completely against the Thai law and was severely offensive to the Thai people ...

The case was eventually dismissed that June, for "lack of evidence" (Bowen's defense was that he had no actual cameras or equipment with him at the time). However, two months spent awaiting trial, sitting in a Thai jail cell, must surely not have been much fun at all.

I sent Annabel the news story of Bowen's arrest and she replied saying she felt he truly deserved it. One widely known fact that emerged from the 1995 event was that Bowen never paid her for it (an amount of some US$10,000) and in her email response dated April 10, 2007, she wrote to me: "How utterly de-lovely! I hope that he will be the fortunate recipient of all the Thai anal action that he has ever desired. I am sure his fellow inmates will be delighted with some plumb white meat to practice their dark arts on."

Following that overseas misadventure, Bowen returned to Los Angeles and still lives there today. He has been married six times – his third wife was the pornstar Misty Regan – and he is currently married to a Filipina. When he was inducted into the *AVN* Hall of Fame in 2001, he gave a long interview to the magazine about his career, explaining how he had formerly been an art dealer who entered the adult business because one of his clients offered him a job art-directing a porn movie that she was financing: "So she offered me a ridiculous amount of money, and I realized then that I was a whore. The movie was called *Miss American Dream*, *Miss American Dreamgirl*, something like that. I remember that Misty Regan was the star of it, and she raped me in the wardrobe room. And I eventually married her."

He started his own company, Fantastic Pictures, which produced and released several Annabel Chong films, including *The World's Biggest Gangbang*. "Making movies is a very big deal," he said. "It's all I care about. When Fantastic Pictures came to an end, I was really devastated. I was a partner in it with *(directors/producers)* Bill Witrock and Chuck Zane. And there were financial inconsistencies that brought that to an end … And after two years it was an unbelievable shock to find there was no money. That left me emotionally scarred for a long time."

That financial insolvency was supposedly the very reason why Annabel never got paid for that gangbang movie. Bone, to his credit, never gave up. He then created Amazing Pictures with Metro Studios followed by the ill-fated Cream Entertainment, and finally, back then in 2001, The John T. Bone Company. That *AVN* interview ended with a quotation that could well be one of most priceless in porn:

I never try to make a bad movie, no matter what the circumstances. Even if there's no money, or I hate the people

I'm working with, or whatever. You still try to make the best movie that you can – and that movie is your life at that moment.

And then you make it and you edit it and it goes out and then it's on to the next one, and you instantly forget that movie. So every one is like the most important thing in my life.

And I barely remember any of them.

Porn, as Bowen was painfully aware, is a quick-turnover business. The final products are often interchangeable, akin to the high-rotation of talent and the musical chairs of partners each actress goes through. Every girl in porn gets her own sexual appetite sated at some point or other, since they're constantly having sex for a living (and, often, not even knowing who they'll be fucking until they arrive at the set – which is, to me, the most erotic component in this strange tableaux).

Veteran porn actress Nina Hartley once told me that people should always remember what porn really is – "disposable, masturbatory material … live action sex cartoons."

Which, in turn, makes things like an Annabel Chong epic in which she's gangbanged 251 times seem … well, almost inconsequential.

* * *

And yet, you could also argue, it was not inconsequential at all.

The event was arguably staged like a "mockumentary" –

mocking the Messalina legend in parody – and the five-men-each-ten-minutes routine might well make it the ultimate live sex cartoon ever made. If it had a redeeming quality that made it meaningful, it was simply this – it was the first time such a thing had ever been captured for posterity, with cameras rolling throughout, and it had therefore acquired a certain sanctity; it had become part of our cultural canon, like any piece of filmed material stood as proof positive that something had happened, something organic and vital and alive.

This argument (which I make in complete seriousness) needs to be seen in the context of adult entertainment. It's a very highly structured environment, which leads to all kinds of desperate behavior as everyone attempts to claim their share of the ever-shrinking pie. Sociologist Sharon Abbott, who wrote her doctoral dissertation at Indiana University on pornstardom as a career choice, noted in a summary paper (entitled "Motivations for Pursuing and Acting in Pornography") that:

For actresses, one means to achieving a career in pornography is to make themselves consistently desirable and available (at least visually) to the public. This includes erotic dancing, modeling, being photographed, granting interviews, responding to fan groups, appearing at award shows and signing autographs at trade shows ... Actresses who display little interest in moving up are often criticized by their coworkers and others as "fuck bunnies," "sluts" or "skags" and are seen as lacking ambition, skills or knowledge. This judgement is encouraged by the assumption that any pretty woman can make it in porn if she wants to. As unskilled laborers, the work of actresses is regarded as fairly easy, even in comparison to their male coworkers, who must "perform" to remain employed. In addition, because of higher pay and higher levels of publicity and fame, females reap more benefits in the industry. Therefore, those who cannot make it despite these advantages are assumed to be lacking personal ambition, with little consideration given to structural constraints.

Yes, it was an industry that did empower women in one specific sense – the women were always paid much more than the men. (Back when I started covering the industry in the mid-1990s, the female pay rate was US$500 a scene while the male rate was $200 a scene.) And women who had ascended to the A-list could choose their movie studs.

But it wasn't always about money. Whatever you might say about Annabel Chong circa 1995, the one thing she did not lack was personal ambition. It takes a fair amount of *chutzpah* to decide that you're going to do something that will quite likely change the course of history, even if it's only within your subculture, and then to willingly participate in a documentary film four years later, one that resurrected the very importance of that event for an even wider worldwide audience.

Think about it – she was born in May 1972 so she was 23 when the big gangbang happened. That's a relatively late career age for most porn actresses in the United States, many of whom start right after their 18th birthdays (so they can be legally employed) and then burn out within their first three years. Not many stay around past the age of 25, and those that do are exceedingly rare.

And so, when John Bowen proposed the idea to her, she probably thought about it for a while before deciding to do it – in part, surely, for its colossal impact on her career but also for her need to make a big statement, one that would ensure her everlasting fame before she had to literally throw in the towel.

Time was running out, and if she had to make that big statement it had to be NOW. (A long NOW, as it turned out – ten hours.) Never mind the fact that there was, at the time, a glass ceiling – in the unspoken hierarchy of the American porn industry, girls who did gangbangs were often treated as damaged goods, seldom making the industry "A-list" – but then again, she probably didn't much care by then. Because she was about being "professional," however ironically so, and about making a seriously radical gender-bending statement.

No matter what anyone thinks of her (or of the gangbang that was filmed), that very audacity was the one true hallmark of her character. And that's what anyone needs to really consider, when considering what happened back in January 1995.

* * *

However, in the run-up to 1999, there were a few facts about her background that now appear more relevant than before, though none of them can be understood out of context. For instance, both her parents had been teachers (or rather, as she told me herself, they were "teaching pioneers in Singapore") and she herself had gone to two of the best, most liberal schools in the country: Raffles Girls' School and Hwa Chong Junior College.

In the Singapore context, Raffles Girls' girls were generally considered brainy and tended to excel academically, and were given to a more liberal curriculum ("I have very fond memories of Raffles Girls' School," she once told me, "I was in that wacky program and we did what we liked. Good times.") Hwa Chong was one of three junior colleges at the time, the first three in the country designed to prepare students headed for university within the British "A-levels" curriculum. Hwa Chong had a reputation for hiring expatriate teachers, mostly from the United Kingdom, who fostered an almost Montessori atmosphere where students were encouraged to discover what they were passionate about and learn things in a much less rigid fashion.

In *Sex: The Annabel Chong Story*, she is seen going back to Hwa Chong and even seeing some of her old teachers, none of whom were aware of her mutation into an adult film star. They seemed like an affable, enlightened lot – a far cry from the kind of teachers I myself suffered under. If Annabel Chong was a product of that kind of liberal, progressive school system and her parents had been teachers themselves, it's quite probable that she always saw herself ahead of the curve. It made perfect sense that she would be a pioneer herself in whatever she later chose to do – she was hardly irresolute in her stern resolve to excel, but only in the best way she knew how.

In one of my favorite scenes in *Sex: The Annabel Chong Story*, she looks straight at the camera and says: "In Singapore, pornography is filth. And that's okay, but it's become a national ideology, a value judgement. To do pornography is to be against the collective agreement of what it means to be a Singaporean. Fuck 'em. They can lick my ass."

We had our own collective agreement.

Over the years, we've had some interesting discussions about the influence of her academic background in Gender Studies. She specialized in modern feminist theory and we've exchanged thoughts about her hero Jean Baudrillard, the French thinker who had posited theories about "simulacra" – simulated versions of reality serving as "modes of mediation" – and we were both very much in agreement with her own assertion that "pornography normalizes sexual behavior through simulacra."

Any study about pornography today, it follows, is really a metaphysical search for Annabel Chong – an inquiry into what she stood for, by way of what pornography itself stands for.

I also shared with her my own thoughts on the people who had inspired my own leanings – like the work of Jacques Lacan (first introduced to me by my friend Anna Span, the British porn director) and the late American thinker Susan Sontag (whose 1967 essay "The Pornographic Imagination" exerted a profound impact on my impressionable young mind back in the day). Susan Sontag had made a point of noting "the disparity between the understated or anaesthetized feeling and a large outrageous event" (said event being, for instance, a gangbang) and Anna Span had quoted this when she wrote her fine-arts degree thesis (on pornography from a female perspective) at London's Central St Martin's College of Art and Design, setting the wheels in motion for her own future career by addressing many difficult issues.

For instance, she addressed "how is it possible to show sexual satisfaction adequately, as an invitation for the viewer to associate him/herself with the characters onscreen ... to represent the physical sensation of the sexual act" so that the character that you choose to identify with somehow acts as an empty body, a chalice for you to step into with your imagination." This, she proposed, involved a process that was actually facilitated by the thin plots and flat acting, without which "you have to use your discursive mind which acts as a lever, separating you from your surrogate body."

I thought that a very important point, indeed – the "discursive mind" and the "surrogate body" being two concepts that made perfect sense from the vantage point of pornography.

Indeed, it would only be many years later that I would come to realize the actual impact of my enthusiasm for Susan Sontag during my undergraduate years (I majored in political philosophy); she was the real *agent provocateur* of my own life, for her writings had indirectly prepared me for my own professional writing career and the bailiwick to come (pardon the pun), as I scrutinized the sex industry in its many forms and guises. And to think that I had discovered her years before she herself had come clean about her own sexuality, including her decade-long lesbian relationship with the photographer Annie Leibovitz (an open secret in the New York arts scene, widely publicized when Sontag's death was reported in 2004).

Well, the intricate connections in our lives are always interesting, aren't they? All too often, we connect easily with our kindred spirits because we all have the same information sources.

That's why it was so easy for someone like Annabel Chong to appreciate where I was coming from. She even told me over drinks one time in Singapore (in November 2006, to be precise, at the Hotel Inter-Continental's Victoria Bar, where not a single person recognized her), that "aside from my mother, you are my only link left to Singapore."

I found that quite endearing, despite how neither of us had ever planned on representing Singapore for *anything*.

* * *

And so, the first thing to remember now is that it was never about the actual setting. The Romanesque production design was meant to reflect the mythology of a nymphomaniacal

Roman empresses who had challenged prostitutes and even worked as one herself. It probably made the poor naked guys standing in line feel like they were part of something important, something historic, something they might even tell their grandkids someday.

But I wonder how they felt after Annabel herself explained it. That they were all actually much less important or historic, compared to the message they were being used for.

The guys wanted to use her as a sperm receptacle and John Bowen used her as his piggy bank. But she herself knew she possessed a sheath for a weapon.

I've always loved the imagery compelled by the very word "vagina" – a word derived from Latin which means "sheath for a weapon."

If the cock is metaphorically a sword, and the vagina its sheath, does the latter in its own way not serve as a weapon in its own right?

Is it not the function of a sheath to preserve and protect, despite repeated thrusts into it?

And wasn't this a symbiotic relationship, since one cannot fully function without the other?

*   *   *

"After the first 100 men or so, you realize the number is just a concept," she had told me. "It's not about sex *per se*, it's about exploring the concept of what sex is. Firstly, it's not sex as intimacy. It's sex as sports. It's public sex. Sex is getting more and more public now. Look at, like, the Calvin Klein ads. More and more, in our society, sex is becoming a spectacle. So how can we draw the line between what we do in private and what is otherwise? That sort of thing, it feeds into each other such that the private and the public no longer is important, and we're moving towards sex as 'information.' How many guys? 251. Or 300. Or 551, whatever, you know.

"And the other thing is the invention of this whole genre, this new genre of sex films that really does not come from the tradition of erotica or pornography but comes from somewhere else, like *The Guinness Book of World Records*, or sports. It's more like sports. There's a historical parallel between gangbangs and orgies and fertility-goddess rituals, but in our society our communal ritual is sports. It's football, soccer, whatever. It's really interesting, this playing out of our modern religion, which is sports."

The way I actually saw it, porn had parallels with professional wrestling. You can actually still enjoy it even when you know it's all fake. The people who had a problem with that were people who were reading it all wrong. If they disliked wrestling because they thought it made a mockery of what sports should be about, they were entitled to that view. But, really, it's not sports at all. It's entertainment.

And porn functioned in almost exactly the same way. "We read the world wrong and we say it deceives us," as the Indian poet Rabindranath Tagore once wrote.

There's an age-old truism that persists in adult entertainment, that sex workers of all levels are presumably glad to be making the most of what they had (selling their bodies, along with their charm and charisma) to get what they needed (the money, the money and the money), but pornstars are unique in that they occupy the only rung on the sex work totem pole where they do what they do because they all have the irresistible urge to perform for the camera. While escorts, call girls, massage parlor specialists and the rest of them thrive on discretion and secrecy, pornstars were the most outrageous of the lot because they wanted to get everything out in the open, for all to see.

I'd heard it so many times from so many pornstars I'd met – "The more guys watching me, the more of them I know are masturbating because they're watching me, the better – that's such a huge rush for me!"

But sexual exhibitionism aside, there was the subsequent conversion of that currency to fame in the public sphere, and that's really what they all crave – mass adulation, the capacity to have your own fan club, the sheer power of knowing that people will actually get in line and wait patiently for your autograph.

Like guys waiting in line for a gangbang.

That's what they all did. That's them grabbing your attention, if not exactly "taking care of you."

But Annabel Chong went one step further. She was in the service of Messalina's revenge, knowing how the nymphomaniacal empress had already transcended her murder. Because they would remember her forever.

Because she hadn't merely captured your attention.

She had captured your imagination.

3

DOUBLE TROUBLE

On March 28, 2009, I received an email from Annabel Chong, asking me if I would go on a trip with her to, of all places, Iceland:

Hey Gerrie!

This is a blast out of the blue, but I have the MOST brilliant idea. I am looking for a travelling companion. Anyway, in the light of Iceland's recent economic meltdown, the krona has fallen to the pits, and I have decided to go on a little vacation to Iceland to take advantage of the exchange rates and to … ummm … stimulate their economy. Unfortunately, everyone I know is either laid off, about to get laid off, afraid to get laid off, or pregnant. Thus, I have nobody to go to Iceland with.

Here are some examples of how insanely cheap everything is:

Hotel: 3 nights at the Hotel 101 (the best hotel in all of Iceland) about US$204 a night.

Food: A gourmet tasting menu at the BEST restaurant in

Reykjavik, Sjavarkjallarin, works out to be about US$45 per person. Tasting menu at VOX is US$65 with wine pairings.

It is also the cheapest place on the planet to buy luxury goods, if you have a sudden urge for Prada.

We can go soak in the famous Blue Lagoon, see the Geysir, go hiking, visit museums, etc. We got 4 days to do that. The plan is to arrive at Reykjavik in the morning and head to the Blue Lagoon from the airport to unwind for a few hours, before checking into the hotel. We will rent a car so we will be mobile.

If we go in May/June, we get 20 hours of daylight. We can thus have the option of going to see the sights at "night" and avoid the crowds ...

Please don't tell me you are pregnant and cannot go.

Cheers,

Grace

Well, I really didn't know what to say to that. I certainly wasn't pregnant, and no former pornstar had ever invited me to travel with her, much less to Iceland, a country with only 317,000 people (120,000 of them in the capital, Reykjavik). We could channel the spirits of dead Viking raiders and marvel at an amazing country run by an openly gay prime minister, with an actual professional comedian presiding over Reykjavik's city hall. This was before its lovely volcano Eyjafjallajokull caused havoc with European airspace, too. It sure was tempting.

I called her and we chatted over the phone. I told her I

appreciated her invitation but I couldn't go. I was then in the middle of working on a book about another pornstar, Monica Mayhem (the book, *Absolute Mayhem*, was eventually published that October) and so I said thanks but no thanks. No rest for the wicked.

She told me she was dead serious about it, and I thought it so nice of her to ask. It brought back to mind something I wrote years ago – "Annabel Chong, over dinner one night, pointed out to me the fact that we were the only two people from Singapore involved in the adult film industry." Those were the opening lines of my book, *In Lust We Trust*, my porn industry memoirs, written back in 2005. Some people at a party I went to in Hong Kong actually re-read them out to me, verbatim, as I stood there feeling quite bemused.

It all harkens to a sense of shared belonging, of spiritual kinship, and the echoes of collective memory.

The truth, however, is that that little factoid hadn't occurred to me until she said so, back in 1999. Unlike today, there were very few Asians in the porn industry at all back then, unless you were of the female, feline, purring porn chick kind. I only knew, at that time, of one other journalist like me who was Asian – my *AVN* magazine colleague Wayne Hentai, but he was Japanese-American and from Hawaii (as opposed to myself, being actually Southeast Asian despite my Southern California accent). We were all such an anomaly in those good ol' days, and I recorded this perspective in the paragraph that followed:

We ate out on wooden deck with a panoramic view of Benedict Canyon, a setting so lush that we could've been in Tuscany but for the howling coyotes reminding us that we were still in Los Angeles. Perhaps it was the crisp autumn air, a nice if nippy chill we'd never get back home, but Annabel thought her observation really funny. From a country of four million people, there were just the two of us. From a country where porn is illegal, no less, which made us an even rarer pair. Double happiness. Or double trouble.

"Double trouble" is how I prefer to think of it, mainly because I had conducted two interviews with Annabel in the wake of the documentary film *Sex: The Annabel Chong Story*.

The first, done on January 21, 1999, occurred as she was heading for the Sundance Film Festival and the timing was perfect, allowing me to explore her immediate thoughts concerning the imminent resurrection of her celebrityhood. The second interview, conducted on March 11, 1999, took place in my car as we drove around downtown Los Angeles. I was then writing a regular column for *Flirt*, a now-defunct website devoting to dating and relationships.

I wanted to do a piece about the fact that the documentary was about to go public, with its impending theatrical release, almost back-to-back like it did at Sundance with another pornstar documentary, *The Girl Next Door*, about a girl from Oklahoma who reinvented herself in Los Angeles as the adult film actress Stacy Valentine. The somewhat odd thing was that I had just interviewed Stacy Valentine herself, which meant all the key issues were still at the forefront of my own consciousness.

Annabel and I talked in my car, while we kept getting lost amid a bunch of one-way streets downtown. I don't even recall where exactly we were even going, to be honest, and if I hadn't switched on my trusty tape recorder that conversation would've been lost forever. Two other conversations about her career also occurred at later stages – one on the balcony of my hotel room at the Regent Beverly Wilshire, where I was staying at the time, and another at the house I was living in, in Beverly Glen Park (the "wooden deck with a panoramic view of Benedict Canyon, a setting so lush that we could've been in Tuscany"). Neither of these were recorded, so the details are definitely lost, but the dinner on the deck was the first time Annabel met my better half, who had been with me six years at that stage (we have been together for 15 years now).

When I asked her some time later what she thought of Annabel, she said: "I thought she was a very regular, normal person – not like a dysfunctional pornstar. Uh, you might not want to quote me on that, since it sounds unfair to pornstars."

* * *

THE FIRST INTERVIEW
The first interview was commissioned by *BigO* magazine, the independent rock music journal from Singapore, and it ran in the April 1999 issue with the headline "Grace Under Pressure."

It remains quite illuminating in terms of how a real person deals with being a celebrity and with the myriad mythologies spawned by her persona – the sheer psychic weight of her own metaphysics.

One of the copy editors wrote a long subhead, serving as an introduction:

You think you know her, but you don't. That's because Grace Quek's porn persona, Annabel Chong, is not just a "piece of meat" who set a world record in 1995 when she had sex with 251 men. Grace's quest is a re-definition of female sexuality, where women can be the studs that men aspire to. And guess what? She was born and bred in Singapore. GERRIE LIM gets this BigO Exclusive with Grace where she speaks of the porn industry, her early years in Singapore, of womanhood and sex, of course.

The preface text I wrote followed, along with the verbatim transcript of the interview. In preparing this section for this book, I listened to the interview again (yes, done on an old fashioned Fuji Type II High (CrO2) Position cassette, a real relic of a bygone age) and made corrections where necessary. The piece ran in the April issue, after the fact – with the Sundance Film Festival being already over – so I pled journalistic license and changed tenses from present to past. In the transcript that follows, I've kept faith with the original version and changed everything back to present tense.

This is how it all reads now – the expanded, warts-and-all version, edited by me:

GRACE UNDER PRESSURE
by Gerrie Lim

The world knows about her now, in all her ragged glory. Annabel Chong is the only pornstar to come out of Singapore, and of late there's been a documentary film about her life, Sex: The Annabel Chong Story, which elicited press raves when it received its world premiere in competition at the Sundance Film Festival in January,

Four years earlier, on January 19, 1995, she'd made history when she set a world record for having sex with 251 men in under ten hours, and the event was recorded for posterity on home video. It's still what she's best known for, despite a career in the adult film industry since 1994 that drew notices for her frenzied carnal antics, in films with self-explanatory titles like All I Want for Christmas is a Gangbang and I Can't Believe I Did the Whole Team!

"Did it hurt? Well, yeah," she told CNN during Sundance. "It's like running a marathon, you know, the pain is part of the high, part of the adrenaline rush." Adding that she likes being treated like "a piece of meat," she takes pains to point out that the marathon crusade was an attempt to subvert the normal parameters of sex, positing questions about the role of women as sexual beings in society while aiming to "explore my own personal sexuality, my boundaries." (In the last stages of that event, she bled from fingernail cuts made by some of the men, and ice had to be applied to her vagina.)

78

Annabel Chong was born Grace Quek, on May 22, 1972 in Singapore, the only child of two pioneering school teachers (her father taught Japanese, her mother music). She spent her formative years at Hwa Chong Junior College and King's College London. One traumatic event possibly triggered her future career – while in London, she got off at the wrong tube station one night and was robbed and gang-raped. This led to her enrolling at the Camden School of Art, where she taught drawing and worked as a nude model, and later at the University of Southern California's School of Fine Arts. She was working on her second degree, a Master's in Gender Studies, at USC when the famous gang bang event took place.

That particular record was shattered one year later, by another pornstar (Jasmin St Claire, who took 300 men to task), but the hype and hoopla had already secured Annabel Chong her place in pop culture history.

The current documentary film, the directorial debut of English-born filmmaker Gough Lewis, charts the path of that iconic status – with some surprising footage actually shot in Singapore. Of Sundance, the film's co-producer, David Whitten, told me that "Grace worked really hard – non-stop interviews from 10 am to 6 pm for seven straight days. She was fantastic. On a scale of one to ten, we hoped she would perform at level seven. She was a consistent ten."

The overachieving lass herself is busy. She's just directed her first feature film, Pornomancer, and is currently creating her own website, which will feature both erotic content as well

79

as an online magazine devoted to "articles about sexuality, politics and art." The interview that follows came about because "I actually grew up with BigO magazine. I've always admired the fact that your magazine offers the alternative voice in Singapore. There's so much censorship in Singapore and I was constantly surprised by what you guys could get away with."

Myself, I'm more impressed by what she gets away with.

Now that you're heading for the Sundance Film Festival, what are your immediate thoughts?

I think Sundance will be quite a hectic experience for me. I'm excited but also anxious, because I don't know what I'm getting into – I've never been to a film festival before, I hear it's going to be a complete circus, so I guess my excitement is tempered by the fact that I have to be prepared to deal with whatever comes up. There is a tremendous interest in the film, which allows me the opportunity to talk about the issues that are touched upon in the film. However, since my interviews are scheduled back to back, I think by day five it will began to feel like a gangbang without the joy of sex! *(laughs)*

Do you have any particular aspirations for the film, now that it's been finished and being theatrically released to the world at large?

I would be very interested to see how this film changes the way people perceive certain stereotypes – certain gender stereotypes

– of the female who happens to be "the other" – you know, the very marginalized figure of adult movie actresses, sex workers, that sort of thing. I believe the film offers a very humanizing portrait. Sex workers are not people whom the general public considers to be human, you know, they tend to read them according to all these stereotypes that have been handed down in mainstream discourse. So I would be very, very interested to see what the reaction to the film will be.

Gough Lewis, the director of the film, met you because he saw you on Jerry Springer, who is perceived as bringing a lot of marginalized people to the attention of the mainstream.
Yes, Gough Lewis approached me three years ago, after seeing me on the Jerry Springer show and reading an article about me in *Details* magazine. It's one of the ongoing debates about Jerry Springer – does he bring marginalized people to the attention of the general society? There's the other camp who says the way he frames them keeps them marginalized. There are the pros and cons about this ongoing debate.

Now, you actually went to Singapore with Gough Lewis to shoot parts of the film, right?
Yes. Initially, when he first pitched the idea to me, I was tetchy. Because there are many documentaries made about the porn industry that are either sensationalistic or exploitative or based on a narrow feminist agenda where all women are portrayed as victims. However, over time, Gough managed to convince me

that his intention was focus on the human side of the subject – "a humanizing portrait," in his own words. On my part, I felt that it's important for a film to get beyond society's stereotypes of the "porn bimbo" or "poor victim," and that by agreeing to do this documentary I would be given an opportunity to address these stereotypes head-on.

There's a scene in the film that's shot in Singapore, where you're walking down High Street, and you turn back to the camera and you say: "Who the fuck do you people think you are?!!"

Right. What is not reflected in the film is the fact that we tried doing shootings at various locations, and almost 80 percent of the time there would be someone coming up and going, "No shooting, no shooting, can't shoot here!" Sometimes we'd call up to try getting advance permission but the moment we got there, they would say: "We've changed our minds. You can't shoot." It's not like an occasional thing – we came up against it every single day. At schools, restaurants, churches, wherever. Even in hotels and stuff. I guess Singaporeans are pretty tetchy about how they're portrayed in the media, like what this bit of footage will be used for.

And the other thing that I really recall from Singapore is this: I went back to my old school, Hwa Chong Junior College, and I was in the bathroom, hooking up my sound gear. I had difficulty getting it hooked up and I was wearing this dress, so the documentary filmmaker had to go into the women's bathroom to help me hook up the sound gear, for fear that I'd completely screw up his sound equipment.

And, of course, someone reported it to the school principal and the story somehow got lost. The event became, "Yes, we saw two naked people in the school bathroom. And the girl was completely naked and the guy was fondling her. And they got thrown out of the campus!" *(laughs)* And after that we went down to Holland Village and we're just having a casual cigarette and taking a break from the stress and two people called my parents, going, "We saw your daughter smoking together with a white man."

But I used to live in Holland Village and it's supposed to be a very cosmopolitan environment.

I know, I know, I used to hang out there. But I guess some Singaporeans have like this thing about the white "buaya" *(Malay for "crocodile")* and those people thought I was some sort of "sarong party girl." So these people called my parents, claiming to be concerned citizens, saying: "We saw your daughter," whatever. But they wouldn't give their names. I found that really funny. It's like, look, if you want to take a moral stance, I respect that, but you should have the courage to say who you are. I would.

Anyway, we had the school principal calling my parents and going, "Do you know what your daughter is doing?" and stuff like that. And it led up to the incident where I "came out" to my parents, and that moment was captured on camera. I thought the filmmaker showed an incredible amount of sensitivity towards my parents in terms of the way they handled that scene because it could've been cheapened into a complete soap opera melodrama. But it was put in such a situation that my parents maintained their dignity. I was very, very grateful for that.

I understand your mother never knew you'd been involved in porn until she was interviewed about you on camera.
I told my mom they were shooting a documentary about me and my life. Because I was doing a lot of performance art, she basically figured they were covering me for that reason.

She thought you were doing it for a USC school project?
No, not that, but we were pretty vague about it. Every single day I felt guilty about not telling her about it. So "coming out" to her was a very good experience for me. We worked a lot of things out. There are a lot of things that I did not tell my parents that I eventually did, and I felt like a better person for it. Because I'm really close to my parents, you know. A lot of people went through complete rebellion against their parents and I never really did. I like being frank with them. So it felt good.

Have they seen the film?
No, they haven't. I plan to eventually fly them over when it's going to be released in Los Angeles. I didn't have time to do

this earlier and also they're tied up in Singapore with some projects that they're doing. I think my mom's doing some music camp type thing. She used to be in the Ministry of Education, planning music curriculum for primary schools. Now she's organizing music camps and stuff like that, and I think she's doing one of those right now. And my dad is in the middle of translating a book.

Would you say they've come to terms with your background and your past, your work in LA and all that?
Well, they know what I do. But, you know, Chinese parents being Chinese parents, it's not something that we talk openly about. They've figured out that I'm fine and I guess they still have reservations about it but they've figured that it's the way I want to live my life. Right now, I'm back in the industry, directing and producing my own stuff. I just directed my first adult feature, *Pornomancer,* for a new company called Impressive Productions, and it's coming out this February. I'm basically directing their entire feature line.

The adult industry is like a micro version of Hollywood, where's there's Hollywood and there's "indie." I'm trying to gear this new company towards the more edgy and more experimental, because there definitely is an audience for that, and that audience is not being addressed. The mainstream stuff is like the adult version of Hollywood, like your average Hollywood movie – tons of budget, looks really good, but nothing ever happens in it apart from a couple of explosions.

I want to ask you more about that in a minute, but first let me ask you something about your education at Hwa Chong. I made email contact with someone who went to school with you. He told me he remembers you being in a humanities class which was taught by a lot of expat teachers. My impression of that is that it probably opened your eyes to what a more liberal education could probably do.

Oh, definitely. I see the radical difference between the regular students who went to Hwa Chong and the students in the humanities program. We were actually encouraged to think and we were encouraged to be critical. Growing up in Singapore, you kind of tend to get brainwashed.

I know, I grew up there myself.

Yeah. *(laughs)* And so these expat teachers, as outsiders, they had a totally different take on it, and it really introduced me to a different way of looking at politics, political systems, society and people.

Of course, within that program, we're geared towards getting into foreign universities. Once I got to England, it gave me enough distance about Singapore to look at it objectively, whereas while I was there I never knew that there was another way to live, that I had choices. By the time I was in my teens, my future was basically plotted out. The way my parents saw it, I was going to law school and I already had a job guaranteed in some prestigious firm. *(laughs)* Actually, it was Lee & Lee *(the law firm co-founded by Lee Kuan Yew)*.

Oh really? It's a good thing you didn't join them. That would've been the end, you know.

I know. *(laughs)* Just thinking back, I realize how radically different my life would have been if I followed the same path that my friends took – the humanities course, the scholarship offered by the Singapore Press Holdings or SBC *(the then-Singapore Broadcasting Corporation)*. They're all doing well, in Singaporean terms. Not all of them are completely happy but, then again, they're doing pretty good. They're getting promotions, they're getting married with children and stuff.

But what really struck me, and made me think twice, was that I had a friend, my best friend from Singapore, she's basically a musical genius – my mom's a piano teacher and we studied and grew up together – and I was the "not talented" one. I had no musical talent whatsoever, and she's really, really talented. And her parents forced her out of it. She got a musical scholarship to go to London, to the Royal College of Music, but her mother wanted her to become an accountant. So she never ever played the piano again.

Wow, that's a shame.

Yeah. Every time I go back to Singapore, we'd hang out and I always felt really sad, because she and her sister, they were really talented, they were the real thing. And Singapore just does not encourage exploration of the arts, although right now it's changing.

Well, that's what they claim.

Right. *(laughs)* I don't really know what's happening in Singapore but they got a pretty good write-up in *Art in America* about the Singapore arts scene, about the edgier stuff like the performance art. I've been out of touch with that and I was just really surprised that all these things were happening. Because when I left Singapore, what was being taught in the art schools was academic painting, what America and Britain were teaching in the 20s and 30s, so it made me decide to pursue an arts education elsewhere.

What are your feelings about Singapore now?

Well – *(pause)* – you know, I hold nothing against it. I don't think Singapore is for everybody. There are people who take well to the system and they seem to thrive on it, and, well, good for them. Whatever. *(laughs)* I do not intend to condemn anybody – I don't think it's my place to do so – but I don't think that it is a system that sits well with me politically. I have a friend who actually entered politics in order to try to change Singapore and, by now, he's like completely given up. Which I was kind of sad about.

We took really divergent paths – he decided to stay and I decided to leave, because I was in a state of despair. I was like, "It's not going to get better, let me just get out of here." He joined the main political party in order to try to reform it from within, but now he's left. He was very disappointed. But I really respected him for trying.

I don't think things are really going to change, at least not in my lifetime.

I don't think so either. It seems that the system is so rigid that people who are able to offer an alternative point of view, they're all leaving. It kind of aggravates the situation and I personally feel like of bad about it. Should I have stayed and should I have fought the system? But it's a no-win situation. I don't see myself succeeding. I see myself getting thrown into jail. It's just a "not my time" kind of thing. But still I wonder.

Well, it's great that you've consented to do this interview for BigO magazine because they're one of the few things there that's still trying to make a difference.

Right. I really respect this magazine. There is so much censorship in Singapore and I was constantly surprised by what you guys could get away with.

Well, it's harder than you think. I did an interview with Asia Carrera and I was told that the publisher was told by the censors that I could not use the word "masturbation."

Masturbation does not exist in Singapore, right? *(laughs)*

Give me a break, you know.

How terrible.

And then, when I did an article about George Michael when he was arrested, I used the word "wanking" and it was okay.

89

What kind of double standard is that?
Right, I know, it's just really strange. My question there is, was it okay because it was a guy doing it as opposed to a girl? Like masturbation in relation to a girl? It still makes no sense. George Michael was caught out because he was cruising, in a gay joint. It's kind of bizarre.

It's very weird. I think they have a long way to go.
Very long way to go. It's hard because I was writing and doing research on gays and lesbians in Singapore, I wrote a paper on it quite some time ago, and I was just astonished. There's an organization – I can't remember the name – but they were trying to get themselves recognized as an official organization and they were turned down and the government refused to give them a reason. So what they did, which I thought was really smart, was instead of forming an organization that's specifically political, they made it a social club. So it was approved.

Have you ever thought of doing your own website?
I'm actually working on it right now. It was supposed to be up on December 15 but because I've been out of town most of the time, I haven't really had time to work on it. It's basically divided into two sections, there's the adult section and there is a magazine section, which is basically free where I have articles about sexuality and politics as well as art. Have you ever seen this magazine called *Richardson*? It's published in Japan.

No.

It's published by these two guys called Richardson and Richardson, and it's really interesting because they kind of synthesize art and politics and pornography but they do it in this really intelligent sort of way. I was fortunate enough to pick up a copy of it from my Japanese friend and I was blown away. There is nothing like it in America. There is another site that I felt was very interesting – I'm really bad at names and it'll come to me in a minute – but anyway the tagline is "literary smut."

Yeah, I know it, it's called Nerve.

Nerve! That's right. They have Norman Mailer and all these people writing for them now. It's really good.

Yeah, it is.

I mean, it's sometimes uneven but I think they're going in the right direction. Where, you know, it can be sexy but it doesn't have to be completely stupid, like the 13-year-old schoolboy *Hustler* mentality. That's what I'm more interested in.

I just saw the book – Nerve is now available in book form.

Yes, it's a collection of essays. I read a review of it and it got a pretty good review.

So what is your website going to be called? AnnabelChong. com?

Yeah, there's going to be *AnnabelChong.com* and the magazine part of it is going to be called *Nero.com*

Nero?
Yes, it's kind of a play on the idea of decadence but it's got a lot of elements of camp. Because if you read about the life of Nero, it's really campy, the way it was retold by the historians. It's just me playing with these ideas, and stuff like that.

Well, I look forward to seeing the website when it's up.
Yeah, by the time I come back in February, I should have more time to work on it.

Your press bio for Sundance says you're interested in exploring elements of sexuality and sexual concepts and you're interested particularly in exploring sex in "regression therapy." Care to elaborate?
I think "regression therapy" was not the best choice of words. *(laughs)* It's kind of a loose concept. It's a big one but let me try to explain.

In psychoanalysis, you're talking about the infantile stage, the pre-conscious, and all psychoanalysis deals with the subconscious, which happens after the pre-conscious stage. And it's in this state where people are polymorphously sexual. According to research, that stage never really goes away. It might remain dormant. If we look at this pre-conscious state, this polymorphously sexual state, if we just look at that concept, what makes it really interesting is that anything could be erotic.

It could be eroticized, and then to take it one step further then, all sex is conceptual. But it's not conceptual in an intellectual sort of way. It still pertains to the body, to the senses, that sort of thing, so from there we can look at social norms and how society determines what is a sexual norm. We take that point of view, that pre-conscious point of view, to function as a critique of mainstream discourses in sexuality.

I know I'm sounding really academic and really stupid and pretentious, but that's sort of like a summary of it. Academic-speak is almost like shorthand, like a secretary shorthand kind of thing, so that's why I decided to use it for that – "regression therapy" – where a four-hour explanation can be reduced to a couple of sentences.

I can see it in terms of an article I read in Penthouse two years ago, about the Jasmin St Claire gangbang. Anthony Haden-Guest wrote the article ("World's Biggest Gang Bang II," Penthouse, June 1997) and it's interesting we're talking about this now because recently, January 19 marked the fourth anniversary of your own big event back in 1995. Now, the point he made was this: After the first 100 men or so, you realize the number is just a concept.

Yes. The number is just a concept.

So it's not about sex per se? It's about exploring the concept of what sex is?

Yes. And what's interesting to me, at least, about this entire gangbang event is that, firstly, it's not sex as intimacy. It's sex as sports. It's public sex. Sex is getting more and more public now. Look at, like, the Calvin Klein ads. More and more, in our society, sex is becoming a spectacle. And so, how can we draw the line between what we do in private and what is otherwise? Could we just be acting out all these media images of sex, where people think that the way they have sex is like – what's that stupid fucking movie, that Michael Douglas and Glenn Close movie? *(pause) Fatal Attraction*! Yes, like they think *Fatal Attraction* is what hot sex looks like! That sort of thing. It sort of feeds into each other, such that the private and the public no longer is important and we're moving towards sex as "information." How many guys? 251. Or 300. Or 551. Whatever.

And the other thing is the invention of this whole genre, this new genre of sex films that really does not come from the tradition of erotica or pornography but comes from somewhere else – the *Guinness Book of World Records*, or sports. It's more like sports. But then, if you look at it again, there's a historical parallel between gangbangs and orgies and fertility-goddess type things. It's ritualized – almost as a ritual – but, in our society, our communal ritual is sports. It's football, soccer, whatever. It's really interesting, this playing out of our modern religion, which is sports. That's looking at it from like a conceptual level.

Well, I think it would be great if we can live in a time and in a society where recreational sex is not looked upon with a kind of stigma, the way mainstream society deems it.
Right.

However, I just read in AVN *that Jasmin St Claire says she's retiring from gangbanging. Did you know that?*
Yeah. That's what she said.

I don't know what your relationship with Jasmin is, but what was your own reaction to her big event in which she beat your record?
Jasmin had her own motivations for doing it and I fully respect it, you know. It's kind of different from mine but, still, she's entitled to have her own motivations. She wanted to basically promote her stripping career and doing something like that would really make her a lot of money in the stripping circuit. So she's made her money and she's a big star now. And good for her. I mean, I have nothing against Jasmin St Claire. I'm actually one of the few people within the industry that she considers to be a friend, whatever the media says.

She's a very difficult young woman, she tends to be bitchy to people and she's actually very insecure. But she's by no means stupid. She graduated from NYU, she speaks four languages fluently. And it's kind of interesting that the first two girls, Jasmin and myself, we're middle-class college students. It's kind of bizarre. I couldn't think of a reason why that is so.

There are now all these people from various areas of the adult industry doing their version of it *(the gangbang)* – there's the gay version, there's the transsexual version, the transvestite version. It's spawned this new genre. Before that, they had this thing called "gonzo" – which was like amateur, *cinema verite* kind of movies, where it's deliberately very raw, with this feeling of "you're there." Really raw, really *verite*. And now this new genre has got a really big following, and now they're churning out a lot of these things or various versions of it.

Do you plan to incorporate this genre into your future work?
I was exploring it on a personal level, as a personal exploration, just to see what it's like. I think what I'm now more interested in is to explore something else, something different. Right now this whole genre is being played to death. Everybody's doing it now. There's no point. It's no longer fun for me to go on beating a dead horse. I want to do more experimental stuff. You know, like, did this film ever make it to Singapore – *There's Something About Mary*?

Yes, but it was cut. They cut out the hair gel scene!
Right. What really fascinated me about that film *There's Something About Mary* – although it's a really stupid movie – was that it addressed this fundamental anxiety that people have about their bodies. Because we live in this really technologically advanced society where it's just really sterile and we live in almost a virtual environment, and

people get really anxious about their bodies. The proof of it is bodily fluids. And I'm interested in how we deal with the unacceptable parts of the body and how it feels to function in socially embarrassing ways. *(laughs)* I think in the next one, I'm going to explore these taboos. That's what was meant in my press bio, when Suzanne Whitten wrote about it as "regression therapy" because it's not longer sex as an aggressive act. It's almost like going back to that messy stage where bodily fluids are okay. It's okay to be a mess! Just get these people in there and we'll shoot a lot of footage and see what happens by leaving it really open. And after that, I can move on to something different. I'm about always moving on, doing different things. As long as I find it interesting, I'll stay in the adult industry. And once I get bored with it, I'll leave. I'm not really interested in having a career. I'm more interested in just pursuing projects that are interesting to me. Because I was brought up to believe that I *should* have a career, and I have been fighting that. And hopefully I will continue to do that unless I'm completely broke and starving. I've starved before when I was living in London but I do not intend to starve again. I'm living pretty comfortable right now and I consider myself fortunate, to be doing what I like and not starve.

On that note, why are you directing now? You have a new film, your directorial debut called Pornomancer.
Well, on a personal level, I come from a background in photography so I've always been interested in seeing what

it's like to direct a movie. Which is totally different and it's got different dynamics. So, I thought, well, by directing adult movies, I could just basically cut my teeth on making movies. And even if I fuck up, it's not going to be that bad. *(laughs)* It's almost like workshop – everything I do and everything I've done is a work in progress, that's the way I saw it.

I met Sharon Mitchell several years ago and I remember her telling me she was directing because she wanted to do something different after years of having sex on camera under someone else's direction. Is that your feeling too?
Yes. I'm sick and tired of starring in these movies that have got the 13-year-old schoolboy mentality. I just wanted to have more control over my material. And, of course, there's this fundamental belief that I could do a better job. I don't know if I can, but I'm going to find out!

What was the experience of directing like for you?
It's a different headspace – I had to constantly switch between "Annabel Chong, performer" and "Grace/Annabel/Whatever, director." Like, "Is the camera in focus?" and "Good, move over this way, I want to get this bit of coverage" and telling people "I want you to get in this certain mood" and "act a certain way" and continuing shooting. So it was like wearing two hats at once, and having to switch personas and states of mind. It was interesting and it was challenging. And then, after that, doing all the pre-production stuff and post-production,

going into editing, cutting the movie together, getting people organized, generally bossing people around and giving them a hard time and being a bitch. *(laughs)* It was a very interesting experience. I probably lost ten years of my life. The first one's always the worst. After that, hopefully, it gets easier.

Do you plan to direct again?
Yeah, definitely. The first time is always the worst because I don't know what I'm getting myself into and I don't know what I have to do. It's about finding it out as I go along. But the second time around, I'll have a basic idea of the process of making it and, in that aspect, it'll be easier. But every single one is different and new problems crop up all the time. A friend of mine who makes films told me: "Filmmaking is about solving problems. As long as you can take it one problem at a time and make sure nothing gets in your way of completing the movie. But be prepared for everything to go wrong." *(laughs)* Which, of course, happened also in the making of this documentary – we met a lot of obstacles. I very much admire Gough Lewis's tenacity. You really have to hand it to that kid. He's really tenacious. Nothing gets into his way. Sometimes he gets depressed and I would be his cheerleader, and tell him, "It's okay, it's all right." Whatever. I'm sure he's very, very happy with the film.

Are you happy with it yourself?
I'm certainly flattered that this young man found me interesting

enough to make this film. And, of course, any documentary will not be a hundred percent accurate, because it's the presentation of an individual, meaning the subject, but still I think he showed remarkable sensitivity and respect – respect to me as an individual, to give me enough space to state my point of view. And of course, the film is his interpretation of me and it's an interpretation that I find very, very interesting.

You seem quite comfortable about using your real name, Grace Quek, again. Do you mind at all having it seen in print?
I don't mind at all. In fact, I like seeing it in print now.

I know some performers in the adult industry dislike having their real names made public, usually to protect their families. You have to understand that Annabel Chong is a persona, she's a character. I think the dichotomy is interesting. I think everybody puts on personas, although their personas may not necessarily have a different name. But now, my parents know about it, you know.

So there's nothing to protect now?
I used to *only* want to be referred to as Annabel Chong before I "came out" so that's the great thing about "coming out," you know, because I can be open about it now.

Let me ask you about Asians in the adult industry. Pornstars like Kobe Tai and Asia Carrera have made some kind of mainstream crossover – Kobe Tai was in the Christian Slater film Very Bad Things and Asia Carrera was in The Big Lebowski – even though they still basically play pornstars in these films. There's some kind of marginalization.

I agree.

And there's also some resistance towards them making a complete mainstream crossover, isn't there? I was just watching the new Metallica video, which had Ginger Lynn playing a stripper, have you seen that yet?

No, I haven't seen it.

I saw it on TV and I thought, "Oh, not a bad video but here we go, stereotyping again!"

That's right. For people within the industry, they're happy enough to get a role in a mainstream film because many of them nurse hopes of making it in Hollywood as an actress. I think it motivates them to take the first role that comes along.

What about yourself? Have you ever been motivated in that direction?

I *cannot* act for like, you know – *(laughs)* My parents were theatre pioneers in Singapore back in the 50s and 60s but I have no acting talent and I'm not about to kid myself. *(laughs)* I have no aspirations to "cross over" as a Hollywood actress, as they say, though I would be interested in doing some sort of weird cameo. Some weird gender-bending cameo where I walk in as a guy, an Asian guy, or something that would be more interesting and funky but does not require a lot of acting and where I don't have to say lines and stuff like that. But, generally, nah, I'm not really interested in being in a mainstream movie.

Do you at least see yourself as a role model for Asians in the industry?

I don't know about that. I don't know if Asians in the industry necessarily need a role model. Because I think most of the girls, the Asian girls I know within the industry, they're pretty sussed. A lot of actresses are on drugs or whatever but the Asians are really together. Asia Carrera, for example, she's a really smart girl, has a shit together, is a really good businesswoman. Minka runs her own fan club. From my experience, the Asian actresses really have their shit together and they have a pretty good sense of where they want their careers to go within the adult industry.

Also, the adult industry is so diverse, just like the rest of society, that the word "role model" does not really apply. I mean, I do not want to posit myself as a "role model" or end up complaining about the responsibility of being one, like Kurt Cobain or Eddie Vedder – an idea that's been so played out. I think there are a lot of people in the industry that I look up to, such as Nina Hartley, who really is almost like a den mother.

And I'm sort of moving towards that direction, playing den mother! People call me up to ask me for advice and I'm always happy to give them advice. If I feel that they're not right for the adult industry, that they have certain things within their personality that will not fit well with the industry itself, I advise them: "Don't do this. It's *not* what you really want to do. It's not for everybody."

Well, I think we all get into careers or end up doing what we do because we have certain questions in our heads that need to be answered, Would you say you've managed to get answers to your questions?

I think a good question is one that demands constant exploration. I think I'm still in the process of exploring the questions I have within myself about my own sexuality and my own motivations. And as I've said, everything is a work in progress. I'd be terribly, terribly worried if I came to a grand conclusion at this early stage of my life. I think it would just be the end of my life as I know it. If I felt that I had answered all my questions in life, I'd have probably gone to law school and probably be at Lee & Lee right now. So, I have no questions that need answering – none whatsoever. I'm happy. I hope that answers your question. *(laughs)*

You told me you were going to meet my former LA Weekly colleague John Powers – did you?

Yes, I did. He left the *LA Weekly* when they changed editors and he moved to *Vogue*, right?

That's right. He was our film editor, when I was at the LA Weekly. What's he doing, writing a piece about you?

No, he's my jungle guide. He's guiding me through the media circus over at Sundance. I consider him a "friend of the film."

That's good. John's a great guy.

Yeah, he gave me some really good advice and he was very blunt. I really liked that. He was like, totally, no bullshit. He was like, "I'm not sure how I should phrase this –" and I'm like, "Just go ahead and shoot, don't be afraid of hurting my feelings. I want to get the lowdown." So we ran through the worst-case scenarios of how vapid things could get and how I could turn certain things back to certain topics that are more, you know, that we felt would be more pertinent to the film.

Yes, film festivals have a weird logic of their own, you know.

Yeah, I know, I know. I'll find out tomorrow. *(laughs)* How strange.

Well, thanks for a great interview. Have a great flight tomorrow and good luck at Sundance! I think this will be a very important premiere for you.

Yeah, I'm very excited.

And you should be!

(laughs) Well, it's good talking to you, Gerrie, we'll definitely

be in touch!
(*Tape ends*)

Looking back now – given the passage of time, the wisdom of hindsight, all that good stuff – I find that while most of that interview was self-explanatory, certain parts stood out as highly telling of where things were in her head at the time. There were also some instances which I found very touching and which were meant for me to hear, in a way that would not have been as deep or trenchant to someone who hadn't also come from Singapore.

For instance, when she reminisced about her late teen years at Hwa Chong Junior College – "Of course, within that program, we're geared towards getting into foreign universities. Once I got to England, it gave me enough distance about Singapore to look at it objectively, whereas while I was there I never knew that there was another way to live, that I had choices."

She never knew that "there was another way to live"?

Most girls her age at the time, if they were going to school in the United States or the United Kingdom, would never have made that kind of statement. Because they wouldn't have had to deal with the heavy indoctrination of the "one look, one style, one choice" paradigm that schoolkids of *any* age in Singapore were subjected to back then.

One could then surmise from that, perhaps, that she had finally outgrown her youthful naivete and, given her eventual career path, surely over-compensated for the perceived lack of choices.

What I've always thought fascinating about Annabel Chong, as a cultural and mythological phenomenon, rests largely on how she took this even one step further – it wasn't enough to merely make an unusual career choice, she had to go all the way and lynchpin it on a conceptual framework, one that was highly surprising for a supposedly bimbotic pornstar. This was the idea of "the number is just a concept" and the fact that "it's about exploring the concept of what sex is" – and how she literally didn't give a toss if people didn't quite get it.

And then, none too surprisingly, she sprung a *caveat emptor* on her fans, the ones who might have cottoned on to her legend for the wrong reasons. ("Right now this whole genre is being played to death. Everybody's doing it now. There's no point. It's no longer fun for me to go on beating a dead horse. I want to do more experimental stuff.")

Well, paradoxically, beating that dead horse turned out to the very game people wanted to play. As recent as August 31, 2010, in fact, when this news report was issued:

METRO MEDIA TO PRODUCE DVD OF SABRINA DEEP 'FAN BANG'
AVN, *August 31, 2010*

Northridge, Calif.— In 2007, Sabrina Deep broke the world's record for the largest gangbang ever broadcast live on webcam when she had sex with 77 men in eight hours. The event was a birthday present to herself.

On Sept. 25, about 40 of her fans will be given their own present: a chance to get it on with "The Queen of the Gang Bang" not only online, when the event is streamed live at FullNaked.com, but also on a DVD that will be released by Metro Media later this year. Deep will invade Southern California for the first time for her latest Fan Bang.

"People have been asking me for a long time to come to Los Angeles," Deep said. "I really can't wait to get into town and get down and dirty with some California boys!" The web star has taken home various accolades, including being named the Booble.com Girl of the Month on two separate occasions (she has natural DD breasts).

Sabrina Deep's World Bukkake Tour has taken her around the world to meet fans. In recognition of this, during a June 2009 visit to The Howard Stern Show, Deep was crowned the Queen of Bukkake. Deep runs her own website, producing 100 percent original content exclusively and shooting with her fans rather than with professional actors.

"My fans are so important to me," Deep said. "Their support and admiration has been what keeps me going. Well that, and their dicks!"

Wow, I thought when I read that, we've gone from Sabrina Johnson (and her 2000-man, two-day gangbang) to Sabrina

Deep (and her 77 men in eight hours), whom I'd never heard of until I read that (but, of course, she's made her point, because *now* I surely have).

Given that Annabel Chong rotated 70 men in ten hours, it is arguable that Sabrina Deep certainly did beat that record. And while there is a conceptual chasm – in my opinion, a fairly wide one – between fucking a motley gangbanging crew (comprising professionally hired studs and amateur volunteers) and fucking your very own fans, you'd have to admire the girl for trying to push that particular envelope.

To me, this also tapped into our own sense of disconnect with what porn or any kind of sex work is – or what its parameters should even be.

However, Sabrina Deep had nothing on my own gangbang girl of choice, the ever enticing Sasha Grey, who at this time of writing can be seen in the latest season of the HBO television series *Entourage*, in which she plays herself. The gangbang genre has really gone mainstream now, and even *AVN* reported on it with a somewhat snide observation, noting that "*any concern over accuracy apparently took a swan dive out the window when it came to the pivotal plot point of Sasha's commanding $200,000 for a gangbang movie.*"

Yes, we've certainly come a long way from the ten thousand bucks promised to Annabel Chong. We *AVN* writers can roll our eyes at that kind of figure, knowing nobody really makes US$200,000 for a gangbang, but most *Entourage* viewers might not know that; they can assume this to actually be true, all because Sasha Grey did this on their hit television show.

So is truth stranger than fiction? The "coming out" of the gangbang as a pornographic device mirrors the original "coming out" of Annabel Chong. If *Sex: The Annabel Chong Story* did one truly good thing, it was this: It humanized Annabel Chong and gave the world a real backstory to rely on. Because deep down, we want to believe in the essential goodness of these girls. (Well, at least I do.) And the fact that the persona she represented, the things she symbolized, had a certain validity and a sense of worth of their own.

* * *

THE SECOND INTERVIEW

I embarked upon the second interview, done on the afternoon of March 11, 1999, as my way of showing her my support since *Sex: The Annabel Chong Story* was about to open theatrically. I'd asked her if I could do a shorter, second interview with her for another publication. She said sure, and suggested we meet for coffee somewhere downtown.

I switched on my tape recorder in the car, with her consent, and we decided to get the interview going while I drove towards a destination that neither of us can now remember.

I don't know why I don't remember it, but I also recall that our meetings were often less discussions than collusions, the kind where kindred spirits meet. Where ideas are exchanged and time flies. I think we were going somewhere for a couple of hours of sit-down and shoot-the-breeze over coffee, something we did every once in a while. The previous time we'd hung out, it was on the balcony of my room at the Regent Beverly Wilshire, back when I was in a hotel and before I moved into a new condo in Westwood. I remember we drank and watched bikini-clad blondes sunbathing below and exchanged porn industry gossip.

This time, in my car, she was carrying with her a book she'd been reading. This smidgen of detail was something I only remembered because, later after I'd sent her home, I found the book under the passenger seat and had to return it to her on the next occasion. The book was *Thing of Beauty* by Stephen Fried – the biography of the 70s supermodel Gia Carangi, one of the first American women to die of AIDS. (The book is less famous than the HBO television movie made from it in 1998 – *Gia*, starring Angelina Jolie, who won the best actress honors at both the Golden Globe and Screen Actors Guild awards in 1999 for that role.)

How apropos, I thought, that she would leave that book behind. I never even told her I'd read it myself, but it seemed like just the thing she would read. At that juncture of her life, she told me she was considering doing outreach work. Dealing with sex workers with their sundry health issues made a lot of sense for someone with her own background.

The interview transcript is, in retrospect, one of the more interesting segments of conversation I've had with anybody. There was a sense of ease and shared intimacy, a kind of honor-among-thieves camaraderie. To some extent, I wanted very much to explore the topic of "celebrity branding" based on what she had told me in the previous interview ("You have to understand that Annabel Chong is a persona, she's a character. I think the dichotomy is interesting. I think everybody puts on personas, although their personas may not necessarily have a different name").

That was said during a more innocent time – if porn can be said to have had innocent times – when a gangbang was as far as you could go. If we see this now, in the context of our present times, that fateful gangbang event of January 1995 heralded the end of an era. Nothing would ever be that simple again, because one year later, the Internet took hold and everyone started downloading and sharing files like there was no tomorrow. "Double-anal creampies" – those certainly didn't exist back then.

I think I only saw my first double-penetration in a 1997 movie, *Fade to Blue,* one of my favorite films directed by the legendary Michael Ninn; that particular scene starred Juli Ashton taking on Earl Slate and James Bonn – made two years after I'd first met Juli Ashton myself (back in 1995, not realizing then what she was really capable of).

Hence my nostalgia regarding the March 1999 conversation that took place in my car. I had also wanted to write about her in relation to another pornstar, Stacy Valentine, who also had a documentary film out that played at Sundance – *The Girl Next Door,* directed by my friend Christine Fugate (the very person, coincidentally, who had inducted me into the porn industry back in early 1995, when she brought me on board to join her team at *Spice*).

The transcript is peppered with hilarious bits of me driving in circles and us getting lost, amid the confusing urban grid of downtown Los Angeles.

Now that you've done the festival circuit and the film is actually about to open theatrically, what are your immediate feelings?
Two things. Firstly, relief that it's probably the end of the entire publicity circus. It's been about traveling a lot and getting heartily sick of it. I guess this is not be the end of it and it maybe might be the beginning of another round of publicity, who knows? Because every time we open a certain city, I'll have to do the local papers and stuff. But it's slowly winding down. It won't be as intense as the year before, doing the festivals and having the nine-to-five barrage of interviews. That part of it is over. The other thing that came to mind is that I don't know how big this is going to be and there's a certain loss of privacy. I don't go out very often but when I go out, chances are that I get recognized. It's a bit nerve-wracking sometimes. Whenever I'm out in public at an event, to a certain extent I'm "on" and it bothers me that people should see me when I'm "off" – when I'm just like dressed in my pajamas and walking around the place. Or when I do not want to be bothered. I really want to believe there's a part of my personal life that does not belong to the media.

But how do you reconcile that? This is one of the problems that comes with celebrity, right? You end up being co-opted into this weird sick fascination that people have with celebrities. How do you reconcile that? Or what have you been learning from the past year that helps you reconcile that?

I think that what I've learned from the past year is to really gather round my close friends. Because they keep me grounded. They are my life outside my job. I really treasure the times I spend with Allen, my best gay pal. Or even just hanging out with David and Suzanne *[Whitten, the film's husband-and-wife producers]* and not discussing work at all. And to be very careful of who I let into my life. I think that was not a concern when I was just "Grace" at the age of 18. But now, it is.

Because of the release of the film – suddenly, all these people, they are now crawling out of the woodwork. They want to get to know me again. They're calling me, they're sending me emails. All sorts of so-called friends that want to do something with me. "Could we work together on this or work together on that?" And I mean, if the project's interesting, of course I would do it. But I deeply resent the fact that people are trying to latch on to me in that manner. I mean, where were they when I was down and out? They weren't there for me. And suddenly, they're like, "Oh my God, I have always supported you!" *(laughs)* Oh well, bullshit. That's disgusting.

Remember the guy from Hwa Chong who wanted to talk to me when he heard I was interviewing you? He was quite cool about it but I was thinking I'm sure you don't even remember him.

Did I go to school with him?

No, you were in another class but he claims he knew you.

Right. Do you know his name?

No. I've got it written down somewhere.

Okay. Because the people that I know outside my class, they're either from the athletics, like the guys I run with, or all the gay guys in school. I was like the gay dating agency. The gay guys would come up to me to ask me who's gay.

Do you think you've got a specific demographic there, among gay viewers or gay people who are interested in the porn industry?

I think it's a generational thing. I think younger gay men will have a tendency to like the film, whereas gay men from the generation that lived through AIDS would have a lot of reservations against it. This is something that came up from my doing the Q&As and talking to journalists. The older gay journalists, they do not approve of the "world's biggest gangbang" because that's what they used to do and –

SEARCHING FOR ANNABEL CHONG

… and look where it got them?

Yeah. *(laughs)* And the younger gay journalists, they were attracted to the politics part of it, to what I say. And also the fact that they could relate to it. It's something that they would like to do but maybe do not have the opportunity or the guts to do it.

Fuck, what are they doing here?!! I hate downtown!

The person who designed downtown should be shot and quartered!

It's such a nightmare. They first time I came down here and saw all these fucking one-way streets, I thought, "Oh my God!" To get somewhere that's two blocks away, you have to circle half an hour. I don't get it. When you live on the Westside and you come down here, it's a whole other planet.

Yeah, I know. It's like me going down to the Valley. I don't often need to go down to the Valley. When I have to go down there for some porn shoot or to interview some pornstars, I get hopelessly lost.

Yeah, that's a whole other planet, too. Do you still do a lot of work for Metro?

No, I don't work for Metro anymore. I used to.

I met James Avalon yesterday, on his set, a Metro film. Did you ever work with him?
No.

I was on his set yesterday because Stacy Valentine was there, doing her last film.
Right. Metro was interested in signing me on but wanted to do my own thing. I decided not to, because if I signed with them it would be exclusive.

Are they a cool company, though, in your opinion?
Yeah, I think they're a good company. They put out a good product, they promote their stars properly, they have a good press department.

The shoot yesterday was amazing. It was in Malibu, actually north of Malibu – Trancas. In Trancas Canyon, inside someone's amazing, luxury house out there. I was there, hanging out with Stacy Valentine and Gwen Summers. And James Avalon and Ron Vogel, who were shooting.
So what does Stacy want to do now that she's retired?

She's starting a clothing line. The girl who designed all the clothes and her wardrobe for her Metro films, September Dawn, do you know her?
I know her stuff, I know her work.

Well, September's apparently her best friend and so she and September are going into partnership together to do a new company with a clothing line, with everything completely designed by September and it's going to be called "Good Girl/ Bad Girl." Well, it's "Good Girl" and "Bad Girl," they're going to be two different lines. They're launching a website to go with the official launch of this company at the end of March – they're having a party at Club Vinyl.

Oh, Club Vinyl! That's interesting. I don't quite know who their market would be, though. I know what their clothes look like.

What do you think of their clothes?

It's not to my taste but, you know, it works very well for porn. I think they would have a following amongst a certain demographic that wants to look ghetto-fabulous. Because they're stuff is very ghetto-fabulous, it's very kind of Lil' Kim-ish, or a toned-down, more streamlined version of it. It's not something that I would wear. What I like about the whole Metro look is that it's not really trashy, it's just porn. It's like glam-porn. All the same, I just don't know who their market would be.

I don't know either. We didn't get around to talking about that yesterday.

I could see a lot of girls who work in strip clubs. They usually go online to purchase their clothing, because it's cheaper.

And they have these mail-order catalogs with all this stripper gear.

Where do you buy your clothes for work?
I make them.

Oh really? I didn't know that.
I make all my clothes. All my feature costumes. If I get them made by a professional, it's going me to cost a few hundred dollars. None of my stage costumes cost more than a hundred dollars. I'll sometimes go to a thrift store to get a dress and alter it and bead it and put on sequins and stuff. Most of the girls wear their little fluorescent stripper gear. What I usually do is, because I'm the feature, I want to look different, so I'll wear lingerie instead. And I don't need to wear their Lycra costumes. For them to look sexy and for them to work long hours in them. But I don't need to work the floor. I stand in the corner and I sign autographs and I take Polaroids, so lingerie works fine.

Hey, do you know what the cross street is?
Huh? We're like right next to MOCA (the *Museum of Contemporary Art*) right now, right?

Sorry. (Still driving, still lost)
I haven't been to MOCA for a long time, too. Shit. We could park nearby and just walk.

Yeah, sure, we could do that, too. I think it's over there. That's California Plaza.
(Her cellphone rings, she takes the call and finishes)

Okay, I need to ask you this – what's your opinion of the Stacy Valentine film? And how do you feel about the fact that your films are opening at the same time?
I think opening the two films at the same time, it's definitely a good thing. Because it will draw more attention to both documentaries. Let me draw an analogy, with *Armageddon* and the other miserable asteroid movie opening back to back.

Yes, and don't forget the two Mars films. You know, Red Planet and the other one –
Oh yes, that's right! The other example could be *Antz* and the bug movie, *A Bug's Life*. When they opened together, they thought that they would be competing against each other. But that's not the case. Because people want to compare and contrast, so they want to go see both. And so I think my take is that it will actually benefit both films, to be opening back to back.

What do you think of the Stacy Valentine film, after seeing it? What's your official comment on it? In 25 words or less?
(Long pause) Let me go off the record really quickly.

Sure. (I switch off my tape recorder, then switches it back on again after she's finished) Yeah, so we can say that, "Debbie Reynolds Does Porn," right?

Yeah. It really is. I really see the film as "Debbie Reynolds Does Porn." Stacy Valentine comes across very well as a sort-of wholesome, all-American girl and she came across as being very, very charming in this very old-school Hollywood sort of way. The sort of perky-blond girl –

… who is totally different from you.

Totally different. And the focus really isn't so much Stacy as herself but it's about following Stacy as a character in the porn industry. So I think the focus is also totally different. It's almost like – let me try to draw an analogy – okay, the only example I can think of is probably *Unzipped*.

The film about Isaac Mizrahi? (Unzipped, released in 1995, was about the development of Mizrahi's Fall 1994 collection.)

It's not really about him. The film's not really about Isaac, you know, it's more about using Isaac to illuminate certain aspects of the fashion business. I'm referring to *The Girl Next Door*, which is more about using Stacy's character to –

– get them inside? Into the porn business?

Yeah. That's right.

Whereas your film is more biographical. It's about you.
Yes, it's more biographical. *(pause)* Do you think that's sufficient for 25 words?

Yeah, sure. David made a similar point last night but I needed this coming from you, to say that you said this.
Right. Cool.
(We reach our destination. Tape goes off.)

The thing that strikes me now about that transcript, having neither heard nor read it for some ten years, is how resolute she already was in her sense of career drive. Steadfast and unwavering from her original goals, she held the line – the film was definitely not allegorical but biographical, she was definitely the antithesis of "Debbie Reynolds does porn," and she was very aware of how that had unexpectedly polarized two generations of gay communities. And she was paying the price of her persona with strangers emerging from the woodwork.

All the attendant hype of the media circus was playing havoc with her headspace and she was making the best out of what could've been a really disastrous situation. Yes, life was nasty, brutal and fragile, but she was taking responsibility for the culmination of what had started out as a whimsical exercise to test the boundaries of her own sexual abilities. In the context of a casual conversation, in which she merely unloaded her thoughts while bring driven around in my car, this was far more poignant than I would have expected.

There was, however, just one small problem.

She was talking to me.

She knew I was no bright-eyed, bushy-tailed ingenue and, more importantly, she knew I was not among the civilians out there who needed to be converted. I was the International Correspondent for *AVN Online*, and was previously the "Cinema Blue" columnist for *Penthouse Variations*. So she knew I was already in her corner, and was transmitting her personal crusade to the outside world.

She was effectively throwing me a challenge: How could (or should) I attempt to be "objective" about the mythology of Annabel Chong?

And the answer is simple. And it's the same one as back then, back in 1999.

I wasn't even going to try.

There's no such thing as "objectivity" when you apprehend any kind of "celebrity branding" – those are not people but "personalities" around whom observers and viewers can build their own sense of psychic affectations. We project whatever we wish onto our favorite film stars, rock stars, even pornstars, all based on what they mean to us.

Sometimes I look back on my own association with the Annabel Chong legend and I think I too had been living my own *cinema verite* "gonzo" movie, where it's all hand-held cameras and spontaneous combustion. I only had to examine the artifacts and relics of the past fifteen years relating to it, while harboring no pretensions to objectivity.

"You think you know her but you don't"?

Of course. And it's still true.

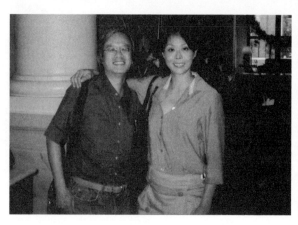

RIGHT
The intrepid author and his unlikely muse – taken at the Hotel Inter-continental Singapore, November 9, 2006. (*Courtesy of Gerrie Lim*)

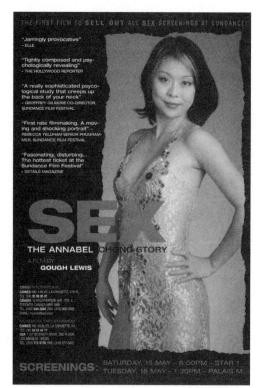

LEFT
"Hot dress, huh?" – the *Sex: The Annabel Chong Story* promotional postcard used for film market pre-sales throughout 1999. (*Courtesy of David Whitten/Greycat Releasing*)

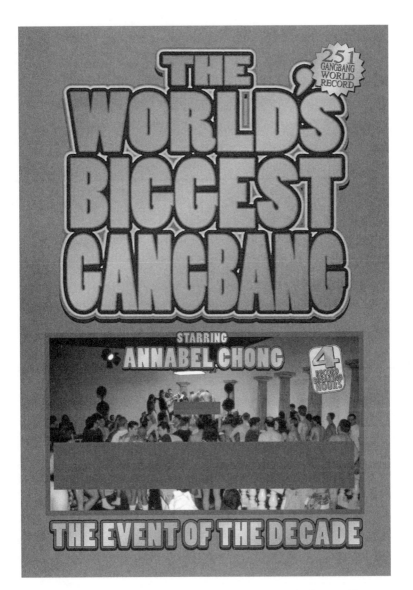

Ten hours that shook the world – the video boxcover of *The World's Biggest Gangbang*, the film that put a certain Singapore girl on the map. (*Courtesy of Metro Media Entertainment, LLC*)

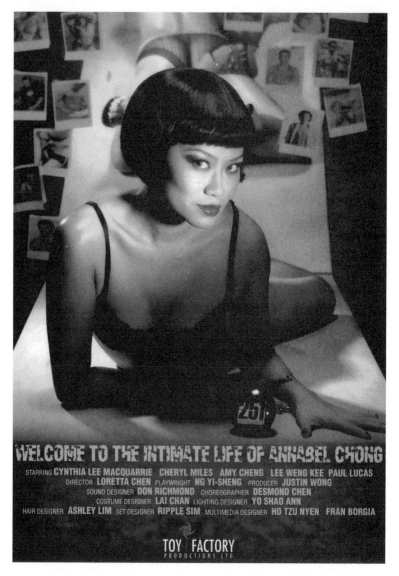

"I am more appalled by the alarming eyeshadow on the actress than anything else!" – as Annabel told me in February 2007, after seeing Cynthia Lee Macquarrie on the *251* stage play poster. (*Courtesy of Toy Factory Productions*)

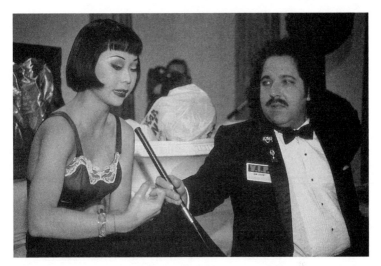

Above "Uh, Ron, you want me to do WHAT with your pogo stick?!!!"
– Annabel with the hardest(-working) man in porn, the legendary Ron
Jeremy. (*Courtesy of Metro Media Entertainment, LLC*)

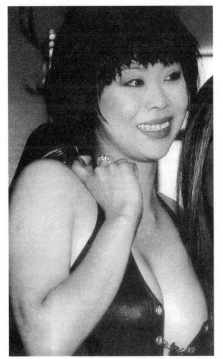

Left Annabel in 1996,
posing with Jasmin St
Claire (standing on her
left, head obscured) on the
set of *The World's Biggest
Gangbang 2*. (*Courtesy of
Zane Entertainment*)

4

ASIAN FEVER

When did the notion of the sexually objectified Asian woman become such a cliche? I remember a house ad that ran in *Hustler* magazine some years ago, for its own Asian-themed sister magazine *Asian Fever*:

Flower Cum Song: Hustler's Asian Fever: This month, give your yang some twang with HUSTLER'S ASIAN FEVER. The sensual secrets of the Orient have been the stuff of legends, fantasies and wet dreams for centuries, from ancient courtesans in flowing silk kimonos to the toddling-sex-kitten styles of today's trendy Japanese girls. HUSTLER'S ASIAN FEVER explores every aspect and every angle of these demure volcanoes of the East with unbelievably explicit photos, stories and illustrations. HUSTLER'S ASIAN FEVER is on sale now at newsstands everywhere. Call 1-800-386-7595 for subscription information.

Now, even I thought that was funny.

What's often less openly expressed is how we have come to accept as normal the many manifestations of this Asian siren stereotype. As Sheridan Prasso concluded, in her book *The Asian Mystique: Dragon Ladies, Geisha Girls, and Our Fantasies of the Exotic Orient*, these expectations emerge from the way Asian women have been depicted in Western culture. "The image of the submissive, subservient, exotic Oriental is a pervasive one: the tea-serving geisha, the sex nymph, the weeping war victim, the heart-of-gold prostitute," Prasso noted. "The actress Anna May Wong once complained that in the sixty films in which she appeared beginning in 1919, she always had to play a slave, temptress, prostitute or doomed lover; whose lines were in 'Chinglish,' who was forbidden to kiss a Western man (illegal until 1948 under California anti-miscegenation laws) and who always had to die so that the woman with the yellow hair could get the white man.

"When criticized for perpetuating stereotypes, she answered that actresses just starting out don't have much choice over their roles. More than eighty years later, the just-as-popular Lucy Liu, when criticized for perpetuating the opposing stereotype gave the same answer – that she did not have much choice, either."

If mainstream actresses didn't have the choices, how could pornstars? All the Asian girls I ever met in the adult business were more than happy to be equal-opportunity sluts. Any way they could get it, any way they could take it. That's the world that Annabel Chong entered in 1994.

Some might call that a perversion of an ideal – of the use of Western ideas in a Chinese context (in Mandarin, *zhong ti xi yong*, the use of Chinese learning for its essence and Western learning for its usefulness) – but to me that's a perversion well worth investigating.

*   *   *

"The adult industry is so diverse, just like the rest of society, that the word 'role model' does not really apply," Annabel Chong said to me in the first interview we did back in 1999. Back then, she was one of the few Asian women who had managed to gain fame beyond her own backyard. The Internet was still young then, and there were not all that many young Asian women who were known outside the adult talent agencies and production studios, in complete contrast to the way things are now.

However, the more things change, the more they stay the same. Today's biggest Asian pornstar, arguably, is the very alluring French-Vietnamese siren Katsuni, who has also shrugged off the "role model" notion. She doesn't even particularly care what her other Asian sisters-in-crime were doing. "To tell you the truth," she told me when I interviewed her back in May 2007, "I don't spend time on the Internet watching Asian girls."

I was asking her about how she saw herself in relation to the other Asian women in the adult film industry, since I figured she was in a rather exalted position and could offer me some valuable insight into the "Asian pornstar" phenomenon, having won more coveted awards in recent years than any Asian woman in the business.

Somewhat to my surprise, she was charmingly dismissive about it. "It seems that scenes with Asian girls are very successful," she conceded. "In any website, it's possible to click on 'Asian' which really proves that lots of men like us. But if you ask me about our sexuality, it seems to me there is no difference between us and other girls who do our kind of scenes."

What she was trying to say was this – there is a distinct difference between what the fans think and what the girls themselves think.

Meaning, many porn fans are often curious, and some even downright obsessive, about Asian pornstars but, at least over in Europe and the United States, the girls themselves don't really care about this racial differentiation.

They're happy to be the recipients of such mass adoration, but the truth is the adult entertainment arena is much too wide for any girl to be satisfied with being a racially defined "niche" performer. You'll never get anywhere in the long run, not if you really want to succeed. And Katsuni, who was previously "Katsumi" (until a name change became necessary when someone also named Katsumi threatened her with legal action), liked her success – but when it's defined on her own terms.

And those terms did not involve her competing with other Asian girls. "There are so many Asian girls now that I really can't pretend to be the best or the prettiest," she said. "I think I'm lucky to be half-French, it brings something special and exotic – Americans love my French accent! Then, it's really about performance, I think. Lots of girls have difficulties doing anal sex but it's really easy for me. I can do rough scenes and I can also act in features. Directors know that I like my job and that I don't complain. Performers know that I do my best, that I really enjoy having sex with them.

"I'm special because I'm just myself, and I bring my personality into my job. If people think that makes me better, I would say okay, thank you, but I'm not looking for competition with the other Asian girls."

I myself believe this to be true: The girls don't believe in competition, even though the fans assume that kind of competition must exist. And the girls don't do so because to do so would mean succumbing to industry typecasting. And nobody wants to be smaller than they should be. They also know that porn is really about representation and variety. I remember reading a sex advice column once where a woman wrote to say she couldn't understand why her boyfriend had failed to appreciate her efforts after she'd given him a home video of herself, fuming that he was bored with it; what she'd failed to realize was that guys don't want a substitute for reality when they watch porn – they want fantasy and variety. And so, the girls in the business supply the variety demanded by the consumer; the more of them populating the business, the better.

When Katsuni did that interview with me, she had just won the *AVN* "Foreign Performer of the Year" award for the *third* consecutive year (in 2005, 2006 and 2007 – no dumb luck, if you ask me, when you're competing with the omnipresent battalions of ravishing Eastern European girls), after already winning "Best Female Performer" in several other porn territories across Europe. ("To win again in the USA means that I really have my place in the X business," she told me. "There are other girls who deserved it but it seems that people really appreciate the way I work, the way I am, and the way I make DVDs sell!")

Annabel Chong never achieved Katsuni's critical acclaim – she won no adult-industry awards at all, in fact – but she also told me once about her own discomfort at being typecast; the submissive *geisha* she most certainly was not. When I asked her about her strip club tours, she gave me some startling information: The majority of her club patrons were Asian, her best stripping markets were Sacramento, San Francisco, Hawaii and New York, and four of every ten emails she received were from fans who were either Asian or Jewish, often about matters academic or philosophical and unrelated to porn.

The fact that Asian guys do flock to watch her, enough to constitute a "majority," merely confirmed my theory. They did have a thing for the Asian girls, but the Asian girls didn't have a particular thing for them.

They were real, *bona fide* pornstars, after all, ready to respond to directions – to fuck *anybody* regardless of race.

After all, that's in the job description.

* * *

However, in the last formal interview we did in the United States, in July 2002, Annabel told me she was "beginning to question to validity of the entire concept of empowerment within the adult industry. Even if one could be a successful entrepreneur, one is still subject to the whims and taste of the fan base, which is rather limiting."

I used this for a *Harper's Bazaar* concept piece called "Bad Girls Made Good," in which she expressed her own need to run against to the grain of the then-popular tide of "bad girl literature" – she had just shelved work on both her autobiography she'd been writing and the planned sequel to *Sex: The Annabel Chong Story* and was about to pull the plug on her personal website as well. She said she "could not understand" the "continuing fascination and sustained interest in Annabel Chong after many years" (to quote her own *Wikipedia* webpage).

So why do the fans care so much when the objects of their ardor often couldn't care less, and where does this kind of parasocial behavior come from?

* * *

Guys get turned on by sexual exhibitionism. It's that simple.

And the exhibitionist herself is exposing her body for anyone to see, caring not a whit who might be looking. She gives in to what sex researchers call the "male gaze" – a term coined by British film scholar Laura Mulvey in her 1975 essay "Visual Pleasure and Narrative Cinema" – Mulvey actually posited two kinds, the "fetishistic male gaze" (where women are seen as "whores") and the "voyeuristic male gaze" (where women are seen as "madonnas"). The good, the bad, and the not always ugly.

My friend Alexis Lee is a walking, talking example of that dichotomy. If young women like her did not exist, I would have had to invent them. (Yes, I know Voltaire said that first, in a somewhat different context, but the essence is very much the same.)

"I enjoyed being watched while I'm taking my clothes off, I really have no issues with that," Alexis (not her real name) told me, before describing a night she'd spent last year at the Torture Garden, a famous London BDSM (bondage-domination/sado-masochism) club. "When the master with the whip asked for volunteers, my hand immediately shot up."

I was sitting with her at a trendy bar in Hong Kong's Soho district. The fact that she was from Singapore made her even more fascinating. She could've been the next Annabel Chong; if not in flesh, at least certainly so in spirit.

"There I was, bent over in front of maybe 30 people, and he pulled my skirt up over the small of my back so everyone could see me," she continued. "It wasn't really a skirt, it was more like a big belt. And I wasn't wearing any underwear.

"I also wore a bikini top with the bra sections cut out, with tiny pasties stuck on my nipples – small enough not to cover the entire nipple area and highlighted with rhinestones to form a concentric circle. As if I needed any more attention called to my breasts! See, I've had this strange compulsion for years, to wear as little as possible without getting arrested. So to be able to expose myself like that, so openly in a public place, was, as you can imagine, a real turn-on for me! Anyway, there I was, bent over, my ass and pussy completely exposed, and the master began whipping me lightly. I could see several guys already jerking off while they were looking at me."

"The master was really skilled with his whip," she whispered. "He kept asking me if I wanted him to stop and I kept shaking my head, no. His lashes were like deep caresses – I had never felt anything quite like it before! There were a few welts that took a few days to disappear, and I remember I couldn't sit down in any sort of normal fashion the whole of the very next day."

I told Alexis I liked her outfit, because she was challenging the viewer to use his imagination when none was actually necessary. That's some postmodern deconstructionist irony for you. And the fact that there were guys in the audience who gave in to self-pleasure (even though the Torture Garden, I was told, frowns upon such behavior), that must have been a thrill for her.

"It was!" she squealed. "You have no idea. I think there

are women who would love to have done that but have never dared to." I can see Alexis smirking now, whenever she remembers that night. *If people back in Singapore only knew*!

She was telling me this, in point of fact, after we had been discussing the work of a porn director we both liked and about what kind of scenes we both enjoyed masturbating to. (When I told her I particularly liked solo-girl scenes, she said, "Nah, I can't watch another girl pleasuring herself without getting banged by a guy. I need to see the banging.")

I'll openly admit I myself was very turned on by what she did in public at the Torture Garden in London. It offered more sexual *frisson* than Annabel's much less spontaneous (and very much more premeditated) gangbang in Los Angeles. I'd written earlier, in my book *In Lust We Trust*, that I had never particularly been a fan of her movies *per se* – "Her style of porn was never my taste – I was not a fan of hard, angry, fast fucking," as I'd succinctly put it – but what I did find admirable was the way she traded in a distinctly unique currency: the shock value of seeing a supposedly demure, telegenically young Asian woman sexually exhibiting herself for all the world to see.

In both Annabel and Alexis, the two kinds of "male gaze" were being put to work. Wasn't shock value a truly cool thing?

That's why Annabel found it easy to catapult herself and her own career with one notorious gangbang event. You may not approve of what she did but she made sure you were never going to forget her for it. Had she declined John T. Bone's invitation, she would probably have remained an obscure Asian pornstar with her own niche, her own small fan base, and spared herself the honor of being the one who called attention to Singapore in the most ironic of ways.

I personally know several Asian pornstars who never did anything that death-defyingly dramatic. In *In Lust We Trust*, I wrote a section about Asia Carrera in which I noted that her example made me realize "why I chose to cover the adult industry, to test to limits of social strictures, like any well-intentioned Asian pornstar would proudly do." Asia was a bright girl, a high-IQ MENSA member, a child prodigy musician who had performed at Carnegie Hall and a scholarship student at Rutgers University in her native New Jersey, yet she gave it all up to be a pornstar.

And she told me she felt very Asian indeed, for her belief in diligence and hard work, and the Japanese part of her heritage gave her a perfectionist streak she was actually quite proud of. But gangbangs just were not her thing, because her comfort zone didn't accommodate that kind of madness.

Mika Tan, an Asian-American pornstar (born of a Japanese/Samoan father and an Okinawan/Taiwanese mother) came my way because of Annabel Chong, who had introduced us. Mika made it clear she had no qualms about working as a legal prostitute at the infamous Moonlite Bunny Ranch in Nevada during the summer of 2009 and she'd even set up an FAQ page on her website to answer questions about it, explaining that she was doing it as a tribute to the spirit of her late Hawaiian-

Japanese grandmother, who had raised her in Honolulu.

"My grandmother was a Madam of several Asian massage parlors," she disclosed. "When the government shut them down after the Vietnam war, she said it was one of the saddest days for her. She felt her parlors were a safe place for men and women to play out their fantasies and, with them gone, men will force their wives to have anal sex, pedophiliacs won't have her school-uniformed whores to role-play, she felt there will be more rapes.

"I agree with my grandmother to an extent. It is my contention that the world will be a better place if people got off every now and then. I am not saying sex is the answer to world peace, but I certainly get cranky when I don't get enough. Ninety-eight percent of Catholic nuns I have met are just plain mean – I rest my case."

To Mika, porn was a much better place than "mainstream" acting, which she had found disastrous. "When I hit 18, I starting going to go-see's by myself and discovered there was indeed a casting couch. My agent told me on more than one occasion: 'Just play nice and see if you get a second read.' My manager once asked me: 'Well, how badly do you want the part?'

"Let me tell you, I learned all my best blowjob techniques trying to make it in mainstream! I know I give pretty damn good ones and if they weren't getting me anywhere, forget it. I refused to go further than blowjobs. I figure, if I was going to fuck for work, I was just going to fuck for work."

Interestingly, I emailed her when I found out about her Bunny Ranch gig through the Internet, and she told me she wasn't interested in talking to me about it unless it was off the record. "What goes on at the Bunny Ranch stays at the Bunny Ranch," she wrote to me on June 10, 2009. "For most of the people here, discretion is everything. I am upholding the Brothel Code of Silence. LOL."

I had another email exchange with her the following day, in which I told her Annabel had expressed disappointment with the newfound vocation. I wrote: "She sent me a note earlier saying she was 'kinda depressed' when she heard you were working at the Bunny Ranch, and I think she would like to know that you're doing all right and that you are fine."

To which Mika replied: "Dearest Gerrie – Thank you for your and Annabel's sympathy, but I don't need it. Good luck with your endeavors. Discreetly yours, Mika Tan." (I didn't share with her a later email from Annabel, in which she wrote: "How is ole Mika doing? Still stimulating the economy? Honestly, I really think Mika could have gotten out of the biz if she really wanted to – she's a smart gal who can get a job at a datacenter as a techie if she really wants to.")

Mika and I had established a bond of sorts when I interviewed her for *AVN Online* in March 2007. She was happy to talk to a fellow Asian person, she told me, since she was "always interested in people talking about the Asian culture – I may speak like an American, but I am still very traditionally Asian. Some people who come over to my house laugh because I am eating fried *Spam* and *kamaboko* on rice with *takuan* and *kimchee*. Regardless of how I am marketed or the crazy roles I play, the person I am when no one is around is someone I am completely comfortable with."

"Is that attractive or erotic?" she rhetorically asked. "I have no idea."

However, she asserted that "Asian women have an awareness of sexuality that is either inhibited or taboo in our Western counterparts. I find a lot of American women to be prudish. Even though many of us Asians do not agree with all the elements of the sex trade in Southeast Asia, we know it is there. We understand how important it is. Whether we know it or not, we all have six degrees of separation from someone working at a hostess bar, tea house, sake bar, happy-ending massage parlor, internet cam site, import/fetish/implied nude modeling. Even though they may not be engaging in sex acts in front of a camera like I am, it doesn't mean that these Asian women aren't marketing sex."

I asked her: "I assume you are most proud of your current fetish work, but a lot of people know of you because of titles like *Ahso's Jap Attack*, *Kamikaze Cunts*, *Krakahoa*, and the very funny *Whoriental Sex Academy* series. I have this theory that it's not an altogether bad thing since those bizarre titles actually lead some people to your fetish work and thereby create long-term fans for you. What do you think? How much crossover do you have between your porn and your fetish fans, do you know?"

"Some of these titles are so crazy!" she squealed. "My fetish fans have very specific criteria. I am not certain a man who likes to see a woman dominate and fuck a man in the ass would be watching me as a Japanese school girl being bukkake'd by five guys."

So she was made of sterner stuff than I'd imagined (I had only seen her straight-porn work, not her harder fetish/bondage work). She also made a comment I really liked: "Do people judge me because I am an Asian woman? If you are implying that they are going to have expectations because of my race and gender, the only thing I can say is I graduated in the top ten of my class, earned a full scholarship, was the editor for the school paper, served as officers for both the student council and the honor society, earned a degree in science, and regularly send money home to take care of my family. Are those the expectations for Asian daughters?

"I just consider myself a self-reliant, strong-willed woman who enjoys sex. I like to try new things and accept new challenges, because you never know when it will be your time to go. So when I die and my life flashes before my eyes, I want it to be a damn good one. Does that make me a role model? People should not aspire to be someone else. They need to find their own way. Their own goals should be what they look up to, not a role model."

But that kind of can-do spirit built upon an attitude of self-determination doesn't sound very Asian to me. Or, at the very least, not the "Asian values" I'd been conned into believing when I was growing up. Where was the correlation between high academic achievement and self-actualized personal ambition?

Mika Tan, like Annabel Chong and Asia Carrera, was an academic overachiever (Mika holds an Associate's degree in psychology and a Bachelor's in biochemistry) who had to discover who she was in her own decidedly unconventional way. How then does anyone begin to judge her, as an Asian woman or as a woman in the first place, in her own right? The very fact that girls were supposed to base their actions of principles different from their male counterparts was the very thing she sought to question, in the first place. It was self-empowerment, done as only overachievers can.

It was in that same spirit that Tera Patrick, the reigning Asian-American queen of porn (who has degrees in microbiology and nursing, incidentally), issued her personal statement of intent on her biography page in the Timothy Greenfield-Sanders photography book *XXX: 30 Porn-Star Portraits*, published in 2004. For my own money, it is the single best career summation made by any pornstar, Asian or otherwise. "Some things in life are choices, while others feel like destiny," she declared. "My hypersexuality, outgoing personality, kink for exhibitionism, comfort with my naked body, and propensity to think outside the box and push the envelope were just a few of my predispositions that landed me in the adult business.

"As a military brat who lived everywhere from Montana

to the Middle East, I was born with a suitcase in my hand. Being half-Thai and a quarter British and a quarter Dutch, I stuck out like a sore thumb – which I thought was a problem until I turned 13 and began modeling for various agencies throughout Europe, Japan and the United States. I learned at an early age that sex was power, and I soon found out that the power was mine!"

Why else do attractive young women become exhibitionistic entertainers, whether they be models or singers or dancers or strippers or pornstars? The sense of being able to control your own destiny though controlling how others partake of pleasure – that must surely be more intoxicating than any drug out there, and infinitely more compelling as a means to an end since it implied complete freedom of choice. The girls always said the same things whenever I asked them why they were in porn – getting lots of sex was good, but not as good as the life choices built into the profession: freedom to choose your hours of work, freedom to travel to exotic places while shooting movies, freedom to transcend the conventional parameters of socially acceptable behavior. And the freedom to choose your own way to make your mark in the world.

It may seem unfortunate to some people that Annabel Chong had to do a gangbang to do so, but the libertarian in me believes she had every right. Sometimes you need unusual methods in order to get yourself heard. Another famous Asian pornstar, Mimi Miyagi tried to so it differently back in 2006 when she tried to run for governor of Nevada. "One-time starlet and Nevada gubernatorial candidate Mimi Miyagi spoke candidly this week with MSNBC about her plans to improve her state's efforts in dealing with increasing growth," wrote Carlos Martinez in his *AVN* news report, noting that Miyagi was "wearing a low-cut, red, white and blue top with a red bow tie that showed off her self-described 36DD breasts." (Choice words used tongue-in-cheek, given her interest in "increasing growth.")

But who really noticed? All that did was add Mimi Miyagi to the long list of pornstars with misplaced political ambitions (a list already hijacked by Mary Carey, Jodie Moore and Stormy Daniels).

What made Annabel Chong different was the way she did it, using the very constructs of porn to make her point. There were surely people outside the industry who didn't know what a "gangbang" was but by the time the news hit in January 1995, a lot of them sure did.

* * *

Once there was a girl named Rose Chan. Born Chan Wai Chang in China in 1925, she grew up in Kuala Lumpur, Malaysia, and became a star on the Malaysian cabaret circuit of the 1950s. At age 27, she was popularly called the "Queen of Striptease" but her career had actually begun in Singapore, where she'd started out as a cabaret dancer at a club called Happy World. She was best known for her outrageous stage acts that included wrestling with a two-metre live python and took her show to Australia, France, Germany and the United Kingdom before succumbing in 1987 to breast cancer at her home in Butterworth, Penang at age 62.

Despite her fame in those countries, Rose Chan remains relatively unknown except to rabid fans of striptease. I myself hadn't heard of her until 2008 when I read that Singaporean director Eric Khoo was planning to make a film about her and was looking to cast a lead actress for the part.

Encountering Rose Chan's existence made me realize how there would always be an interest from sundry quarters about Asian women who made a living from the expression of their sexuality. More than any other racial group, it seemed that Asian women had a stranglehold (especially in Rose Chan's case, given the live pythons); somehow, from the male viewer's perspective, they added zest and zing to the voyeur's tableaux for seemingly contradictory reasons – on one hand, they were working against type (since good Asian girls weren't brought up to be striptease dancers, let alone pornstars) while, on the other hand, they were sometimes reinforcing it (*Memoirs of a Geisha*, anyone?), playing straight into the obvious commodification of gender.

But when you get Asian pornstars who can actually talk intelligently and thus accomplish infinitely more than merely explode the porn bimbo stereotype, you get almost a new paradigm shift in sexual consciousness. Mika Tan told me she was "so impressed" with Annabel Chong after meeting her for the first time, through a photographer who had shot both of them many years ago. How funny, I thought, since some people outside the adult industry would probably see them meeting as one *geisha* specimen meeting another, not realizing that both of them actually held each other in high regard for their intellectual prowess and professional drive.

*   *   *

THE THIRD INTERVIEW

In July 2002, I conducted my last formal interview with Annabel Chong, for the aforementioned "Bad Girls Made Good" magazine piece. I sent her questions by email and here's how the conversation went:

What's your opinion of the current attention being paid to books by women in the sex industry – notably Lily Burana's Strip City and Tracy Quan's Diary of a Manhattan Call Girl as well as Xaviera Hollander's Child No More?
I think it is very much in line with the whole subversive-chic thing that we talked about a few years back. The liberal media is constantly looking for exotic, edgy material, and within American culture sex still provides a *frisson* of danger.

Are you still working on your autobiography?
No. I realized that what I really treasure right now is my privacy, and I do not feel the need to rehash my life for profit.

I am focussing on starting a new life in IT and find satisfaction in being a non-famous, behind-the-scenes sort of person. I actually have turned down most interview requests, because I am sick and tired of rehashing the same statements over and over again for the benefit of the press.

Do you feel a sense of sisterhood with Asian pornstars who are empowered sex-positive feminists? Like Asia Carrera, who also does her own website and runs her own business from it? And, if so, does this bond run deeper for you in any way because you're also Asian?

Yes and no. I deeply admire Asia Carrera, and I applaud what she is doing. However, I am beginning to question the validity of the entire concept of empowerment within the adult industry. Even if one could be a successful entrepreneur, one of still subject to the whims and tastes of the fanbase, which is rather limiting. That being said, I think we need more Asia Carreras in the industry, as they are good role-models for women who work in it. I feel pissed off that people continue to think that she is just a pretty bimbo, and I think the porn press do not give her enough credit for it.

What kind of feedback did you get from appearing in the Los Angeles Times Magazine as a golfer?

My liberal friends think I have sold out to The Man, which I have, and I love it! Actually, most people do not recognize me in that article.

Do you think the "mainstreaming" of pornstars is an enduring phenomenon? It was reported yesterday that Jenna Jameson just got herself a two-book deal with Regan Books/HarperCollins and she's also appearing in an ad campaign for Ikea, the Swedish furniture store! Do you see yourself as part of this trend or do you aim to capitalize on it in any kind of mainstream, commercial way?

I think the "mainstreaming" of pornstars will continue as long as it sells products. However, for every Jenna Jameson, there are thousands of wannabe B-girls who continue to toil from shoot to shoot. They continue to be looked down upon by the mainstream, despite the fact that they are the foot soldiers of the porn industry. Very often, the mainstream would take on a few "token" pornstars, just so it can say, "Look we are so edgy, come buy our product so you can be edgy, too!"

As for capitalizing on my notoriety, I have to admit that it holds little appeal to me – I find it too limiting. I am determined to pursue a career as a private citizen, get my Oracle qualifications and polish up my coding skills. Eventually I would like to get into database administration and software development. Pursuing fame is a double-edged sword – it may bring more money and adulation but at the same time you are confining yourself to a public persona that is subjected to the whims of the consuming public. I personally find that tiresome after a while, having to play the same role even after I have evolved into a totally different person. I have had my little ride, fame-wise, and it was interesting while it lasted, but I think now it is time for me to try something new, something where I get to use my brain for a change.

What is your current status, work-wise? Are you still producing that website as well as running your own site? Are you still dancing on the road? Any more plans to direct movies or complete part two of your documentary?
I am in computer boot camp right now, but I still manage to find time to take on web-design projects here and there, and also run my own website. I am not really motivated to complete the documentary, as it seems too much like backsliding into my fame-hungry days. I am gearing up for my Oracle exams and doing tutorials on coding languages – C++, Java, VB – on my own every day. I have set up my own hybrid network consisting of four PCs and one Mac, and I spend all day on it. I am running Windows 2000 Server as my OS, with Active Directory configured, and my personal database runs on Oracle. Don't tell Larry Ellison.

I love this stuff, and I see it as my ticket out of having to look pretty to make a living, which I hate because I am a tomboy at heart. I think my teenage rebellion is over, and it is time to open a new chapter in my life. In any case, I am getting too old for the shenanigans of my salad days, and I look forward to a boring Republican lifestyle consisting of stocks, golf and home improvement projects.

* * *

Well, did she sound like a good ol' Asian computer geek enroute to being a software development entrepreneur or what? Because that's the route she chose and the road she's still on today. Talk about self-principled self-determination.

I particularly liked what she said about her kinship with other Asian pornstars and how they all were at the mercy of their Asian-fetish fanbase, singing to the tune of *Hustler's Asian Fever* "Flower Cum Song" and living in the long shadows of the famous courtesans of yore. Some critics might even argue that Komako, the fictional geisha of Yasunari Kawabata's famous 1956 novel *Snow Country* had been a more profound expression of the fragile dignity of the sex worker than anything written in more modern times (with apologies to Mika Tan and her VCA film *Memoirs of a Modern-Day Geisha*, made in 2006).

Even in the Japanese AV adult-film scene, there is a curious disconnect. While Japanese society is actually far more tolerant of its pornstars than most others, their AV stars usually only attract mainstream attention when they became sensational news items. For instance, when one of the industry's most successful stars, Ai Iijima, died on Christmas Eve 2008 under mysterious circumstances, it was those very circumstances that were the actual news.

Was she, as some people speculated, murdered? (She'd received death threats, some said.) Was she herself an AIDS patient (which would have explained why she had been such a passionate AIDS-prevention activist), and died from the AIDS medication she'd been taking? There was some talk of kidney failure caused by such medication. In the end, police investigations in 2009 concluded she had died from pneumonia, with no suggestion of foul play.

Ai Iijima, who had also worked in porn under the so-very-sassy name Ai Candy, was a former nightclub hostess and *enjo kosai* ("compensated dating") escort before she became a full-fledged adult film star and bestselling author (her "semi-autobiographical novel" *Platonic Sex* was made into a movie of the same name in 2001). She was apparently dead for almost a week before her body was found in her 21st-floor apartment in the Shibuya district of Tokyo. Amazingly, she had fans who only knew her from her mainstream television-hosting appearances and advertising gigs (she was a spokesperson at one stage for the Yoshinoya beef-bowl restaurants), who hadn't followed her previous Japanese AV-porn career at all, which only made her death even more sensational.

Another example of such media transcendence was AV star Saori Hara, who was revealed in news reports in September 2010 to have been the former Mai Nanami, a fledgling mainstream movie starlet and sometime bikini model – she'd changed careers in 2008 with little fanfare until some nosy reporters put two and two together (since her breasts looked unusually large for a typical Japanese girl).

I only learned this by accident from a Japanese science-fiction website, in a report about the Japanese cult movie *Reigo: The Deep-Sea Monster Vs the Battleship Yamato*, in which Mai Nanami was the lead actress. The startling, newly uncovered (pardon the pun) career change was the news itself, along with an amusing factoid – despite her newbie status among the porn ranks, Saori Hara and her better-known AV compatriot, the Eurasian beauty Maria Ozawa, were now reportedly the two most downloaded adult stars in China, and this in turn had led to Saori Hara being given one of the two female leading roles in Hong Kong producer Stephen Shiu's new film *3-D Sex and Zen: Extreme Ecstasy*.

And so there were, apparently, several ways to get yourself out of the porn ghetto. Saori Hara was luckier than Ai Iijima (who basically died before she was noticed outside Japan) but it always seemed that to get yourself known outside the porn world, you had to be known for something newsworthy that transcended the narrow confines of adult entertainment. Unless you did that, you were only defined by your porn fan base, which doesn't really expect a lot out of you outside the prerequisites of the profession.

Sure, as blowjob specialist Inari Vachs once told me, after she'd won the "Best Orgasmic Oralist" award from the XRCO (X-Rated Critics Organization) in 2000: "It's a hard job but someone has to blow it." But what if you're not satisfied with being known for just that one talent? Sudden deaths and radical career changes were only two ways to transcend your limited sphere, but perhaps the most suitable method of reining in your own madness was to do a very Asian thing indeed – take the money and run.

That's what Annabel Chong did, at least in principle. The money didn't quite come in from the gangbang, but the idea of making it helped eject her from the porn sphere and finally parachuted her to mainstream safety. And however ironic it all must seem now, it was really the smartest thing she ever did with her life.

5

CHUCK PALAHNIUK
LOVES VERONICA LAKE

As the philosopher Bertrand Russell once noted, "One should as a rule respect public opinion in so far as is necessary to avoid starvation and to keep out of prison, but anything that goes beyond this is voluntary submission to an unnecessary tyranny, and is likely to interfere with happiness in all kinds of ways."

Interfering with happiness? I know something about that. For the past decade and a half, I've amassed a collection of files, all relating to the cultural phenomenon that is Annabel Chong – representing so many points of view, reflecting just how complicated a phenomenon she is. There's our email correspondence, our past conversations and interviews, the pieces I wrote on her, the pieces she wrote herself, and the biggest chunk of all: newspaper clippings and magazine tearsheets, stuff written by other people.

This whole shebang started up when I was about to

interview her, right after they announced the participation at the 1999 Sundance Film Festival of *Sex: The Annabel Chong Story* – "they" being the film's producers (David Whitten and his wife Suzanne) and Sundance was, of course, the fulcrum for my lever, the wellspring from which this whole crazy journey began.

In an attempt to make sense of all this, I divided the gigantic mess of press material into three separate files, respectively entitled "Sundance," "Singapore" and "All the Other Crap."

And when I look at these files now, I'm sometimes at a loss as to where to begin.

That's may sound strange, given how short the pornstar career of Annabel Chong actually was. She started working in the adult film industry in 1994 and officially retired in 2003, when she posted a message on her own website declaring "Annabel is dead." Those nine years, however, did not run consecutively – she left porn in 1996 to focus on finishing her USC Gender Studies degree, graduating in 1998, and came back to porn just before shooting the documentary, having also attended the 1998 World Pornography Conference where she talked about her new interests in academic research.

That same year, she started performing as well as directing, and continued to work sporadically. But she had all but stopped performing since 2000, appearing only in a few fetish-oriented videos, and was seen mostly online through her then-new personal website, *annabelchong.com*. The bulk of her onscreen hardcore work was already done and dusted – from

1994 to 1996 – and all the bits and pieces since her eventual "comeback," if cobbled together, amounted at best to a further year or two.

That's maybe four years of actual work over a nine-year period, which is not all that unusual in the adult-film industry. Most girls spend the bulk of their non-filming time going on the road, performing at strip clubs across North America, and Annabel did her fair share (and told me some stories about those times that I can't repeat here, having been sworn to secrecy). Three to five years of "club dancing" time is the norm, for most twentysomethings in porn valley.

So, given how terribly *average* her actual porn career was, it's somewhat astonishing that she generated the amount of press that she did. But the explanation isn't hard to find – the historic gangbang of 1995 received some much-needed help from the documentary in 1999. Were it not for *Sex: The Annabel Chong Story,* her legend might well have passed into obscurity.

In a parallel fashion to say Bruce Lee and James Dean – who both made only three films each but whose legend is writ large indeed, towering over many others with longer filmographies – the mythology spawned by the tandem workings of the gangbang and the documentary made possible a disproportionate representation of her persona, both online and offline.

I went to *Google* for "Annabel Chong" and found 1,340,000 results, slightly less than half of that for "Jenna

Jameson" (3,720,000) or "Sasha Grey" (3,240,000). That's more than what I myself would've expected, given there was never a bestselling book (in Jenna's case) or hit films and television shows (in Sasha's case) to boost the ratings. The reigning Asian-American porn queen, Tera Patrick, still gets 2,190,000 results on *Google* but she's also had a book out and is still active – as opposed to someone who'd retired back in 2003 with no new product of any kind released since then.

But, as Tera Patrick herself pointed out so candidly in her book *Sinner Takes All*: "We're all 'hos on this bus, whether you're a pornstar, a prostitute, a stripper, or a girl dating a rich guy who buys her things."

When you work in the realm of the "floating world" – the demimonde of commodified, commercialized sex – the trade-off is usually much the same, with slight differences of degree. Any way you parse that paradigm, there's that ever-nagging question that stubbornly rakes its manicured nails on your exposed back: How much of your soul did you sell for your measure of deserved notoriety, itself disguised as stardom?

Selling your soul is a by-product of selling your body in adult entertainment, no matter what form that sale takes (even if virtually so, *vis a vis* online downloads or more old-school, still-wankable video movies), and for all pornstars the trade-off is accepted as *de rigueur* – because the hotter and nastier you are, the more visible you will be.

And visibility is *everything* in this business.

154

*   *   *

When perusing my own gigantic Annabel Chong files, I've noticed certain pieces that stood out more than others, in each of the respective categories. In the "Sundance" section, for instance, the best-written assessment of the documentary came from Paul Fishbein, then the editor-in-chief of *AVN*, who took it upon himself to write a comparative study of the two pornstar flicks making their respective marks at the 1999 festival.

His piece, "From Sundance to Cannes: Adult Documentaries Score High Marks" (*AVN*, August 1999) looked at how the Annabel Chong film stacked up against the Stacy Valentine film *The Girl Next Door*. Proving that adult film magazine editors aren't always the been-there, done-that jaded cynics most people might have expected, Fishbein declared that he really, really liked the film and accordingly wrote:

Both films are dramatically coherent, probing and honest, with similar insights into the adult business ... While both Annabel Chong and Stacy Valentine come off as fragile and insecure, Chong is the sadder subject. It makes Sex: The Annabel Chong Story a more chilling portrait. Bright and well-studied, Chong is more than a bit fatalistic. "I believe sex is good enough to die for," she says when her best friend Alan, a transvestite, warns her about HIV. She moved to Los Angeles because, "if there's going to be Armageddon, I want to be in the center of it." Sometimes lucid, sometimes confused,

155

she's a living contradiction. One minute, she's describing a triple-penetration or performing an extreme scene in Depraved Fantasies 3, the next she's involved in a "presidential debate" at Cambridge University.

Sex does an effective job of juxtaposing the two lives of Annabel Chong and Grace Quek. For example, she seems quite uncomfortable negotiating with Robert Black a price to do sex scenes that include fisting and pissing. In the next scene, we find she's an accomplished painter. She spews freely about her exploiting her own sexuality in explicit terms, and describes her entrance into the adult business by saying, "I finished fucking everybody. I had an existential crisis."

Her trip to Singapore (a camera captures a family dinner but parents have no idea why they're being filmed), where her mother finds out about her career and talks about retaining dignity, is as devastating a scene as in any Hollywood drama. When she cuts her own arm just to feel pain, or revisits the place in London where she was once gang-raped, her tortured soul is clearly in view ... And without doubt, Sex: The Annabel Chong Story *is one of the more insightful documentaries on any subject filmed in the last few years.*

It's always great to get a thumbs-up review from *AVN* (I know so, because they did the same for me when my book *In Lust We Trust* was reviewed in the November 2006 issue) but that one took me somewhat by surprise – Fishbein was so quick to point out the key elements that mattered. Only someone with enough years in the business would have zoned in on such hilarious soundbites, like "I finished fucking everybody. I had an existential crisis."

For pornstars are often born of existential miasma. I could cite quite easily the young women I met in the business who had told me about how, before they got into porn, they had "fucked half my dorm in college" (Juli Ashton) or how "I had been a teenage runaway who exchanged sex for room and board, so getting paid to do porn was actually a step up for me" (Asia Carrera).

The "existential crisis" is about what to do next – after you've sold your body enough times for free, you might as well sell it for money. As one pornstar, Dyanna Lauren, once told me about her own life, having left the highly exploitative, ethically challenged music business for the relatively more benign porn business: "I decided that if I was going to get screwed, I might as well get paid for it."

There's always a ready market for existential pain.

When Fishbein calls Annabel a "living contradiction" who exposes her own "tortured soul," he was zoning in on the very elements of the Annabel Chong persona that made it a marketable brand. *Details* magazine also noted this in its own Sundance roundup: "Far more provocative and disturbing than any porn-doc yet made," wrote Mark Ebner in its April 1999 issue. "Two revelations made the doc even more fascinating: Chong admitted to sleeping with director Gough Lewis during the making of the movie – and revealed that Lewis even marked himself with a razor blade after Chong had cut herself onscreen. 'He was so moved by it that he joined in,' Chong said. We've heard of getting close to your subject, but this is scary."

Score one for the triumph of shock value, though I'll bet he's pissed off at the scars today.

The other pieces in my "Sundance" file illustrated other key facets of the Annabel Chong legend. Many of them were offshoots of the piece circulated by *Agence France-Presse*, the French wire news agency, which opened its report this way:

FAMED SINGAPORE-BORN PORNO STAR ANNABEL CHONG A SENSATION AT CANNES

by Jocelyn Zablit

Agence France Presse

May 21 1999

One of the more unusual movies Korean buyers snapped up at the Cannes Film Festival this year is the story of Singapore-born Grace Qek, who gained world fame in 1995 by having sex with a record 251 men in a 10-hour period ... The film deals in blunt terms with why an intelligent and well-spoken middle-class student of fine arts at the University of Southern California would seek to have sex with 300 men in order to set a world record, until then held by an Amsterdam sex worker.

"Annabel Chong is a persona I created to express a certain part of myself that so far has not been able to find an outlet," the 26-year old Qek told AFP. "In some ways Annabel is a rebel, she is rebelling against her very strict

upbringing in Singapore."

She said though she had initially picked 300 of the 1,500 men who applied for the porn exploit that was captured on film, she decided to stop at 251 due to fatigue and because she had to complete a university assignment for the next day – a "book review on bisexuality."

"It's unfortunate that the American media does not realize the humor in the 251 event, which is supposed to be an over-the-top parody of what men are supposed to be like – you know the idea of a stud who just wants to (sleep) with anything that moves," Qek, who speaks in a mixed British-California accent, said. "It was aimed at denouncing the male quantitive approach to sex."

She spelled her last name wrong but, to her credit, Zablit summarized the key selling point of the Annabel Chong mythology – her ability to articulate ideas relating to her own self-expression of sexuality, itself born of disaffected youthful rebellion, and the very admirable charm offensive that came with it. She had a certain panache that made people sit up and question their assumptions about the "porn bimbo" archetype. *The Straits Times* in Singapore on May 23, 1999 ran an abridged version of that AFP story next to a photo captioned: "Looking shagged in Cannes was Singapore-born Grace Quek aka Annabel Chong, who was promoting her film *Sex: The Annabel Chong Story* on Thursday."

There were several other snippets from the press coverage from snowy Park City, Utah that year, which saw 118 films shown (70 of them world premieres), and I've singled out these for special mention:

From Andrew Strickman ("The Films to Watch at Sundance, *MSNBC*): "Sex: The Annabel Chong Story – Without a doubt, the single hottest ticket entering the festival, this documentary from director Gough Lewis trains its eye on Chong, a 22-year-old Master's student in Gender Studies, who had sex with 251 men in one 10-hour day, under the aegis of research."

From Paul Clinton (*Turner Entertainment Report*): "'Did it hurt?' Well, yeah. It's like running a marathon, you know, the pain is part of the high – part of the adrenaline rush. It hurt, but it's not something I didn't expect' ... This is the same woman who speaks in the documentary of being flattered that so many men wrote in wanting to take part in the marathon: 'If that's not an ego trip, I don't know what is' ... 'What I hoped to accomplish, firstly,' she says, 'was to explore my own personal sexuality, my boundaries, and I think I accomplished that. To see how far I could go off the beaten track of the passive female who likes to be romantically seduced' ... 'Don't you think,' she says, 'that by putting women on this terrible pedestal, where they're all pure and perfect, is kind of terribly constraining on women? It really puts this terrible limit on what they can do in life. It's just another way of controlling – limiting the avenues of exploration that women are allowed to do.'"

From Rebecca Yeldham (*Sundance Film Festival 1999 Film Guide*): "Cliches define female pornstars as typically deluded and self-destructive, victimized by the patriarchy that controls the industry and consumes its product. Such stereotyping assumes a state of disempowerment that Annabel Chong, an unrepentant, self-styled feminist defensively denies. For Chong, pornography is a vehicle by which she can exert her will, sate her rampant sexual cravings, and assert her repugnance for societal repression and the "politically correct" constructs of sexual normalcy. But as the camera probes behind the rhetoric and hollow stare of its feisty protagonist, we begin to piece together the complex mosaic of Chong's inner nature and the troubled history that informs it."

From Jeffrey Wells ("Sundance Confidential," *Mr Showbiz*): "The film is being shown five times at the festival. Exploitation? Titillation? No way, says Sundance topper Geoffrey Gilmore. He calls it a "really sophisticated" psychological study that "creeps up the back of your neck" ... Annabel – Grace – spoke with us last week from New York, where she was working briefly as a stripper to pick up some extra cash before flying to Park City ... 'I'm not interested in being politically correct,' she says. 'I'm more interested in being interesting.' She says she submitted to the gangbang 'to see how far I could push myself sexually. Sex is not just a private act. It doesn't have to be about intimacy. I think it can also be a sports event. Sexuality is a terribly subjective thing. Some prefer monogamy and some prefer something different.' Grace counts herself among the latter ... Grace speaks with a guarded tone. A lot of women in the sex industry have a hard time relaxing or opening up with the press. And we don't want to sound unkind, but we feel there's a truth-in-advertising problem in the selling of Gough's documentary. Despite all the hype (not to mention the copy in the Sundance program) Chong didn't actually have sex with 251 guys. It was more like '70 or 80,' she says. 'We recycled them.' This raises all kinds of questions that we'd rather not go into."

Ah yes, such are the things that make up our iconic cultural figures – the metaphysics of hurt, the "troubled history" that makes for "psychological study," leading to the "questions that we'd rather not go into." The waters are made murky when deception is revealed, and some people must have theorized that it was perhaps her own bad karma – that she deserved to not get paid for the endeavor since it was a cheat and a lie, with the studs being "recycled" so that 251 "acts" became misconstrued as 251 "men."

Does a penetration make a man? Wasn't that the very thing she was questioning in the first place?

There are two diametrically opposite ways of seeing this. One posits that any kind of penetrative act constitutes sexual activity, regardless of the instrument used (which makes sense, since "solo-girl" scenes in porn often involve a lone pornstar self-pleasuring with a vibrator), while the other disputes this and insists that unless it happens to be a penis at work in a sustained fashion, it really shouldn't count as sex at all. (And Bill Clinton's cigar didn't count either.)

Ask the girls themselves – all pornstars know it's not what

you use but what gets you going. ("Sex is anything that gets you down here," Vivid Video contract star Cheyenne Silver once said to me, running her own palm between her legs and rubbing her crotch slowly, giggling as she did this.) Taking the woman off the pedestal by way of consensual degradation then makes perfect sense in this context. Polymorphous sexuality blossoms when any act can be sexually fetishistic. She was extolling the virtues of more open-minded thinking through a seemingly grotesque act committed in full public view via the technology of home video.

The problem, though, was that a lot of people just couldn't see past the grotesque nature of such a sensational event. Nobody really cared about the ideas behind it.

So who's fooling who now? Hadn't people forsaken the message by shooting the messenger?

*   *   *

It took some doing but I eventually made a shortlist from the items in my "All the Other Crap" file, and these were the ones worthy of closer scrutiny:

"World's Biggest Gang Bang II" by Anthony Haden-Guest (Annabel is mentioned *vis a vis* Jasmin St Claire's own gangbang event of 1996), *Penthouse*, June 1997.

"So Many Men" by Emily Jenkins, *Mirabella*, September 1999.

"She's Faking It – You Can Tell: The Annabel Chong Story

Sucks" by Bret Easton Ellis, *Gear*, July/August 1999.

"Seven Inches of Pleasure with Annabel Chong" by Rosy Ngo, *Pop Smear* magazine, September/October 1999.

"Voice: An Interview with Annabel Chong" by Amy Goodman, *Nerve.com*, 1999.

"The Child Defiled" by Gary Morris (an opinion piece about Annabel Chong), *Bright Lights*, July 2000.

"Sex: The Annabel Chong Story" by Pym Pernell (news report), *AVN*, March 1999.

"Annabel Chong's Biography" (from the Excalibur Films website, January 1999).

Luke Ford's mini-biography of Annabel Chong, from his own website.

"Practice Makes Perfect' by Leslee Komaiko (Q&A interviews with four amateur golfers including "Grace Quek, 29, writer, Hollywood"), *Los Angeles Times Magazine*, August 5, 2001.

Snuff by Chuck Palahniuk (in which Annabel Chong appears in seven of its 197 pages), novel published in 2008.

There would have been a twelfth item, but its importance was ironically diminished by the achievements of some other pornstars. The March 1995 issue of *AVN*, the "*AVN* Awards – CES '95 Wrap Up" issue did report on the January 1995 Annabel Chong gangbang but it was apparently deemed not important enough to merit a cover story – instead the cover featured then-rising VCA Pictures contract star Juli Ashton who would, a few years later, be re-signed by VCA to an unprecedented US$25,000-per-film deal (more than twice what Annabel would have made for the 1995 gangbang). Three other pornstars appeared on that cover, in smaller photo insets following their respective victories at the 1995 *AVN* Awards – Asia Carrera (who had just won the coveted "Best Female Performer" trophy) and Kylie Ireland (who had just won "Best New Starlet") seen posing with the legendary Tiffany Million.

Well, it was a busy business constantly rife with competition, so perhaps the timing was wrong if they'd wanted an *AVN* cover. (The *AVN* Awards are always held in January, so John T. Bone might have known better than to schedule his gangbang shoot that same month.) Trade journal stories tend to be self-congratulatory, anyway, so it's more instructive to consider other sources for serious analyses of the Annabel Chong legend.

Anthony Haden-Guest's June 1997 piece for *Penthouse* was really the first one that drew my attention to the whole gangbang phenomenon. "Way back in 1991, a woman had taken care of 125 men in Norway," he observed, "and Annabel Chong, a lithe young person with black bangs like the actress Louise Brooks, had doubled that figure in 1995. Jasmin St Claire was now proposing to accomplish 300 men, thereby exploring the do-able limit, the wear-and-tear equivalent of an under four-minute mile."

"In cool point of fact, though, one suspected that the *Guinness Book of Records* people were not holding the printing presses for the result," he added. "'Three hundred' was a concept, rather than a number. Indeed, I had spotted several individuals performing, then rejoining the end of the line and going up for seconds. I pointed this out to John T. Bone, a laid-back fellow with a gray beard, sandals, and a diamond stud in his ear. It came as no news to him. 'Some are going up for thirds,' he said, adding meditatively. 'Does that constitute a relationship?'"

Haden-Guest then interviewed Jasmin St Clair after the cameras had shut down:

"Why didn't you go to 325?" she was asked.

"If you had 300 cocks in you, you wouldn't want to go to 325. Trust me," she said with some edge to her voice.

* * *

AVN redeemed itself four years later, with Pym Pernell's short news item, arguably an attempt to correct previous editorial oversight. As befits a trade journal that should be appropriately supportive, it adopted a rather sympathetic tone.

"Anyone in the mood for a good documentary? No? Well, you might change your mind when *Sex: The Annabel Chong Story* is released sometime this year," is how the report starts, noting that it took Annabel three and a half months of talking with Gough Lewis before she agreed to do his film, with the film's debut at Sundance taking place three years after she'd first been approached about it.

"The biggest misconception about me before people see

the movie is that this is a film about a porno chick who is supposed to be this out of control hyena," she is then quoted as saying. "I hope that the film would complicate people's basic assumptions about women in pornography, the representation of women in pornography, as well as the nature of female sexuality."

That single quote remains central to my own study and the word "complicate" is essential towards my own analysis. Porn is a complicated subject and people's own assumptions about it are oftentimes too simplistic – because what most consumers tend to believe are often based on egregious errors, half-truths and sheer hyperbole. Like the "biography" on the website of Excalibur Films, a major adult movie retailer:

Annabel was born on May 22, 1972 in China. She was educated in Singapore before moving to England as a young lady. Annabel's sexy English accent adds a spicy twist to her striking Oriental good looks, making her one of the most exotic women in porn. Upon her debut in the porn ranks (in a great scene in More Dirty Debutantes #37), Annabel wasted no time in showing herself to be one wild, insatiable sexer. She is one porno starlet who it can be said specializes in gang bangs, having appeared in lots of kinky gropes for (John T.) Bone. Her sweaty tussles in flicks like I Can't Believe I Did the Whole Team! were just a prelude to her starring roles in the four-hour marathon World's Biggest Gangbang, where she took on more than 70 men in a fiery, tiring sexual adventure.

Annabel doesn't always need to be in a gangbang to sizzle, though, as her top-notch erotic performance in Voyeur 2 with Jon Dough and Joey Silvera proves. She's a kinky, crazy sexual dynamo who is one of the most popular Asian porno stars ever.

That was the first time I saw it written that she had been "born in China" (Singapore sounded like it could've been in China, for all anyone cared) and the choice verbiage certainly contributed to her complaint about being perceived as an "out of control hyena." Prescriptive descriptions like "one wild, insatiable sexer" and "kinky, crazy sexual dynamo" did sync perfectly with many male consumers' perceptions of pornstars. She had, in her movies, all the frantic, fast-fucking moves to justify those, too.

That's why, in complete contrast, the *Los Angeles Times Magazine*'s golf interview was a deliciously funny counterpoint to all this. The exchange took the form of a quickie questionnaire:

What kind of golf day are you having?

Above average. I had a really bad one three days ago.

How long have you been playing?

About four and a half months. But I play every day.

Do you have a favorite club?

Probably my 7-wood.

What would your nickname be?

There's the Tiger. So I guess I'd be the Kitten.

The interviewer, Leslee Komaiko, knew how to milk this

for what it was worth, despite factual errors (There's no such golf club as a 7-wood – she must have meant "7-iron" or was attempting irony with a sexual metaphor). "Blame it on Tiger, but golf driving ranges are busier than ever," she began her piece, noting the interviews were all done at the Rancho Park Golf Course, a two-level range with 43 slots on the more affluent Westside of Los Angeles.

The irony of "Blame it on Tiger" would have been far more apparent today, of course, but even then his reach as an inspirational figure was awesome to behold. And I really like her asking to be called "The Kitten" (as a playful turn on the "sex kitten" role, even when she wasn't named as Annabel Chong.)

Luke Ford's "bio" of Annabel on his website, on the other hand, was quite a different kettle of fish. An Australian based in Los Angeles, Ford was previously a male model and aspiring actor who, as he once told me himself, experienced an epiphany one day while mulling his then-struggling career. He decided the best way to achieve much-needed fame and acclaim was to start a website devoted to the porn industry, whereby he could transform himself into a gunslinging gossip hound and pull no punches, with the express aim of exposing the sundry goings-on in the San Fernando Valley.

This, unfortunately for him, did not always translate positively, as he found when one pornstar sued him for writing that she had sex with animals and several other prominent producers and directors sent him warnings (and the occasional

occasional death threat) merely because he had written about them in ways less flattering than they would've liked.

It was in this can-do, devil-may-care, gung-ho spirit that Ford wrote of Annabel Chong, posted on January 19, 1999 (the fourth anniversary of the original gangbang event):

In 1995, Annabel Chong got banged 251 times to set the world record. Seventy men showed up to do Annabel repeatedly until she was bleeding the last couple of hours and ice had to be applied to her vagina. Poking fingers with uncut nails cut her up.

Ron Jeremy boffed all five fluffers before finishing Annabel off.

To find men, Annabel advertised on videos and in magazines that she wanted men to fuck her. Her invitation read: "I'm looking forward to meeting you – and eating you." Hundreds of men sent in photos of themselves but only 70 showed up. Some requested anonymity.

Annabel got screwed out of her $12,000 pay which was supposed to cover her USC expenses. Her parents ultimately came to her tuition rescue. Chong says she'd forgive Chuck Zane for not paying her if she could fuck him up the ass with a big dildo.

AVN *comments that Annabel should learn from the experience not to screw 251 men on a handshake.*

Ouch! But it actually gets worse. In a section about her adult film career (not written in chronological sequence but rather in Ford's typical zig-zag manner that pays no need to syntax or style), he contended that:

The star of Anal Queen, Sordid Stories With the Pink Stiletto and I Can't Believe I Did the Whole Team says making X-rated films is great for someone as sex-crazy as her.

Like many performers, she'd rather skip the complexities of dating. "I don't need to go out on a date and be nice to someone to get laid," she says. "I can just fuck, take a shower, and go home. People have called me a bimbo, a slut and a whore. But I just enjoy my body."

Unfortunately for Annabel, many porn users don't enjoy her body. She's not been in much demand since her record breaker. Her appearance suffers from lousy dental and boob jobs ... After completing her sex marathon, Annabel said she wanted more. "Two hundred and fifty guys isn't enough. I could do with a few girls too – and a few dogs and cats."

In Annabel's first day in porn in 1994, she gangbanged seven men.

Annabel believes herself to be a "conceptual artist" ... "That was totally gross," says Kia. "She got $10,000? How much is that per guy? Fifty bucks?"

Luke Ford may not be the world's best writer but it was almost a neat touch that he quoted another Asian pornstar, Kia, in a manner that implied prostitution with a sick twist. (The quote is slotted in from out of the blue, since Kia is not mentioned elsewhere in his text!) He was groping to score a point without seeming opinionated, if rather clumsily, and that theme (*"How much is that per guy? Fifty bucks?"*) elevated his report to the level of farce.

And farce was the exact device adopted by satirist Chuck Palahniuk in his novel *Snuff*, itself a parody of the porn industry. The American author from Portland, Oregon was already no stranger to sexual candor, having already achieved a formidable reputation with novels that specialized in postmodern irony – he's best known for *Fight Club* and *Choke,* both made into good movies – and his novel *Haunted* featured a famously ugly masturbation scene (famously so because more than 200 people fainted during his readings on his 2005 book tour to promote it).

Snuff goes all the way by showcasing the adventures of pornstar Cassie Wright in her attempt to set a new gangbanging record with 600 men. Palahniuk openly acknowledges the trailblazing example of Annabel Chong, who appears in the book by way of providing both context and subtext, as the following gems illustrate:

When Annabel Chong set her early record … performing 251 sex acts, even with eighty men showing up for the cattle call, some 66 percent of them couldn't get their dicks hard enough to do the job.

Gang bang protocol, ever since Annabel Chong first called the shots, it says all the guys have to wait, schlong-out naked, Ms. Chong, her fear was some crazy with a gun or a knife. Some Holy Roller, hearing direct orders from God, would answer the casting call and murder her.

Ms Chong's best skill was crowd management. It was her

idea to bring the men onto the set in groups of five. Among those five, the first man got erect was the one got to screw her. Each group was on set for ten minutes, and whoever was able got to ejaculate. Even if some guys never got hard, never touched her at all, all five counted toward the 251-man total.

The real genius was to make it a competition. The erection race. Plus, studies show that when males are placed together in close proximity before a sex act, their sperm count will rise. These studies are based on dairy farms, where bulls will be staked in groups near a fertile cow. The resulting harvest will yield greater volumes of viable semen. Stronger convulsions of the pelvic floor, maximizing the height and distance of the expelled seminal fluid.

Want to talk third-wave feminism, you could cite Ariel Levy and the idea that women have internalized male oppression. Going to spring break at Fort Lauderdale, getting drunk, and flashing your breasts isn't an act of personal empowerment. It's you, so fashioned and programmed by the construct of patriarchal society that you no longer know what's best for yourself.

A damsel too dumb to even know she's in distress.

You could cite Annabel Chong – real name: Grace Quek – who fucked that first world's record of 251 losers because, for once, she wanted a woman to be "the stud." Because she loved sex and was sick of feminist theory portraying female porn performers as either idiots or victims. In the early 1970s, Linda Lovelace was delivering exactly the same philosophical *reasons behind her work in Deep Throat … Do you respect someone's right to seek challenges and discover their true potential? How is a gang bang any different than risking your life to climb Mount Everest? And do you accept sex as a form of viable emotional therapy?*

It only came out later, about Linda Lovelace being held hostage and brutalized. Or how, before becoming a pornstar, Grace Quek had been raped in London by four men and a twelve-year-old boy.

Early adopters love Annabel Chong. The damaged love the damaged.

Megan Leigh shot more than fifty-four films in three years and then bought her mom a half-million-dollar mansion. Only then did the star of Ali Boobie and the 40D's and Robofox shoot herself in the head.

Isn't a kid alive who doesn't dream about rewarding her folks, or punishing them.

Annabel Chong compared a gang bang to running a marathon. Sometimes you felt full of energy. Other times you felt exhausted. Then you'd get your second wind and feel your energy rise.

Once she became empress, according to the historian Tacitus, Messalina fucked gladiators, dancers, soldiers – and anyone who refused her, she had them executed for treason … At the time, the most famous prostitute in Rome was named Scylla, and Messalina challenged her to a competition to see who could couple with the greatest number of men in one night. Tacitus records that Scylla stopped after her twenty-fifth partner, but Messalina kept going and won by a wide margin …

All this I told to Ms Wright as we sat in my apartment eating popcorn and watched Annabel Chong fuck her way through 251 jizz-juicers. Groups of five. Ten minutes per group. Sock-soakers. Bone-beaters. The set decorations, the white fluted columns and splashing fountains, a historical creation of Messalina's challenge to Scylla. The fake marble and Roman statues. The World's Biggest Gangbang. A student in gender studies at the University of Southern California, with a grade point average of 3.7, this film was Chong's tribute to Valeria Messalina.

The part about Megan Leigh (who committed suicide at age 26 in 1990) was deliberately, and perfectly, placed. I doubt it's that easy to generalize – all sex workers get into their profession for a whole host of reasons, often too complicated for quickie psychoanalyses (Megan Leigh started out by working at a massage parlor in, of all places, Guam!) – and I myself wouldn't claim that Annabel Chong, as an extreme form of angst-ridden rebellion, was a deliberate attempt to punish her parents. But it opens up the debate, and might be plausible if viewed from an Asian-centric perspective – suspiciously so, since she was an only child – though from a more Western-centric stance it's a lot easier: Just blame it on Messalina.

In the final analysis, Palahniuk is probably fairest to her among all the observers in my files. The instances where she appeared in *Snuff* were quite likely factual – at least the "crowd management" thing was her own idea, we know that for sure – but I also thought it intriguing that the best representation of her turned out to have emerged from the sensibility of a novelist, somebody who writes fiction, and a writer of satire and farce, to boot. I thought this quite fitting, since Palahniuk clearly *gets* it – because he chose a jaunty, playful tone of voice to reflect Annabel Chong's own playful notions, aimed at getting people to be less serious and uptight about sex and, by proxy, empower them to discover their own sexual comfort zones.

Palahniuk once said in an interview that he was very fond of a line uttered by the 1940s screen siren Veronica Lake: "I wasn't a sex symbol. I was a sex zombie." (Raymond Chandler, who wrote the script of her film *The Blue Dahlia*, once called her "Moronica Lake.") So, like he did with his earlier (and better-known) novel *Fight Club* with its theme of repetitive violence, he was really asking in *Snuff* one pointedly sardonic question.

Can you push your own sexuality to an extreme edge, like getting banged in a gangbang, and still respect yourself in the morning?

* * *

Note to reader:

Chuck Palahniuk wrote, in an email to me dated December 14, 2010, about his novel *Snuff*: "I want to stress that the tone of the narrative voice I used does not honestly represent my own view. While the world-weary character making the cited statements might seem to disdain Ms Chong, I, myself, have nothing but the fullest respect for her. In time I hope the gesture she's executed is recognized as a culture-changing milestone in the evolution toward gender and sexual equality."

6

SINGAPORE REBEL

I t's always interesting to see how a famous person is treated
back in their own home country. Are there people in Cuba
who secretly love and revere Gloria Estefan even though she
had long defected and had become an American in Miami?
I don't know for sure (and neither does Gloria herself, quite
likely) but I do know that Annabel Chong has many admirers
back home, and some detractors too, many of whom make
no secret of how they feel. And all these views hinge on how
she is supposedly representative of the notion of rebellion
in Singapore, which until recent years was a notion much
frowned upon.

Case in point: In 2007 I was asked to serve as a consultant
on the stage play cleverly called *251* (bearing the slogan:
"Welcome to the intimate life of Annabel Chong"), which
opened at the Esplanade Theatre in Singapore on April 5, 2007,
produced by the Singapore theatre company Toy Factory. The
play's director, Loretta Chen, wrote to Annabel through me
seeking Annabel's blessing to do the play and felt she needed

to explain to her the motivations behind her effort.

Loretta, who has kindly agreed to divulge parts of her letter to Annabel, wrote that she had "always been fascinated by Annabel – less for what she did, than what she stood for."

"A lesbian feminist myself, I was educated in Singapore and then went to London and the U.S. for my postgraduate," she told Annabel in the letter, "so I always did understand this sense of awakening that happens when one leaves claustrophobic Singapore. I was gripped by how petty and how small-minded we were in Singapore and questioned our hypocrisy and attitudes towards sex, homosexuality, religion, the works.

"Anyways, to cut the long story short, I wanted to play devil's advocate to our government's constant appeal for entrepreneurs, notion of the 'can-do' spirit and question just where we drew the OB (out-of-bounds) markers for the definition of a national hero. The papers were abuzz with news on local athlete Khoo Swee Chiow scaling Everest and diving to deepest waters, etc., and I wanted to then ask what a local hero was. It seemed to the press that one was considered a hero if he or she broke records and dared to do what few would do – Annabel hence came quickly to mind.

"Why wasn't she a hero, then? Because her act was sexual and because she was female? That seemed like an interesting angle as it was almost a fatal loophole in our collective psyche. Thus 251 was born, as I really do want us to take a step back to examine our own hypocrisy, projections, double standards.

And maybe I really just wanted people to begin to love and understand Annabel Chong the way I thought I did when I watched *Sex* – I cried with her at the end ... I wished more people saw that film as it gave insights to the person behind the persona."

In the end, ironically, Loretta's very touching letter of spiritual invocation turned out to be better than the play that resulted, which in my opinion failed to reflect her ambitious intentions.

* * *

Singapore's main newspaper, *The Straits Times*, hasn't featured the country's only internationally known celebrity all that much, but there have been a few notable mentions.

In a big feature on September 13, 2006, regarding the publication of the 640-page book *Singapore: The Encyclopaedia*, reviewer Ong Soh Chin mentions her – "HIV/AIDS is listed in the book as is porn actress Annabel Chong, the Singapore girl who really was a great way to fly." An accompanying piece by book reviewer Stephanie Yap noted the glaring omission of the book's own editor-in-chief Tommy Koh (formerly Singapore's ambassador to the United States and also the country's representative at the United Nations) – "This, despite the fact that other Singaporeans, like ex-pornstar Annabel Chong, made the cut."

She then quoted Tommy Koh explaining his own omission,

saying he felt conflicted about it since he was editing the book, though he pledged that "no entry was left out for political or moral reasons" and he was "determined to maintain objectivity and balance." Koh also said, about the inclusion of Annabel Chong: "We had a long debate about whether or not to include her. The more conservative members did not want to. But in the end, we felt she deserved an entry as she had achieved a certain level of notoriety."

Two respected *Straits Times* writers, Ignatius Low and Colin Goh, penned pieces that were fine examples of armchair philosophy – Low's was entitled "Doing the Unthinkable" while Goh's was called "Prodigy or Tragedy?" and both addressed the real issue at heart, the sheer damage done to the psyche of most Singaporeans thanks to years of a dysfunctional education system coupled with an achievement-crazed social system.

What that kind of system eventually produced was, arguably, an angry creature called Annabel Chong.

Colin Goh, who wrote a lively Sunday column in the paper, used his soapbox that day (April 6, 2008) to discuss the issue of post-traumatic stress in "gifted" children, taking as his starting point the scandalous story of Sufia Yusof, a mathematics prodigy who went to Oxford University at age 13 but was later found working in London as a prostitute. Goh wrote:

I find Sufia Yusof's story tragic but I can't say I'm entirely surprised. I had the same feeling some years ago when I attended the New York premiere of a documentary on, perhaps, Singapore's most famous gifted student: Grace Quek, better known as Annabel Chong.

For those of you unfamiliar with Ms Chong, she rocketed to worldwide notoriety with The World's Biggest Gangbang, a pornographic video of her having non-stop consecutive sex with 251 men (later revealed to be actually "only" around 70).

"Annabel" turned up for a post-screening Q&A session, which I thought she fielded deftly, and I was left with the impression of someone extremely smart, but so full of hurt and rage that she felt compelled to respond in an extreme way ... While watching the documentary, I remembered thinking: How uniquely Singaporean of her not to be content with just making porn, but trying to break a record while at it.

I'm not suggesting in any way that the pressure of excelling academically automatically leads to risky sexual behaviour, but I do think that growing up in artificially constructed circumstances can mess you up.

That last sentence rang true. Achievement-oriented societies naturally produce people obsessed with breaking records, though I think Annabel Chong actually did more than merely break a record – she actually broke a barrier. If nothing, her greatest achievement lay in making more than a few people rethink their preconceived notions of conventional "vanilla" sexuality.

Ignatius Low and I engaged in a lively email exchange after his "Doing the Unthinkable" piece was published on November

13, 2005, mainly because I liked his piece a lot. While similar to Colin Goh's in being sylistically first-person philosophical, Low had one distinct advantage – he was actually a classmate of Grace Quek at Hwa Chong Junior College for two years, and so her personalized his piece by bringing up his memories of her:

My first impression of Annabel was formed on the second day of orientation. A small crowd had gathered on the school field where she had pinned another classmate of mine – the son of a permanent secretary, no less – to the ground. Four- and seven-letter expletives flew as she threatened him. And all he had done, if my memory serves me right, was sneak up on her unawares and soak her with a homemade "water bomb."

I remember being amused and yet in awe of her. And these mixed emotions returned many times over the next two years.

For although Annabel was brash and attention-seeking, she exuded the sort of confidence that took your breath away, whether it was radically interpreting poems in literature class or talking back to our expatriate tutors.

Although her antics sometimes came across as foolish, she possessed a type of daring I often wished I had. So I've ended up vicariously basking in the attention that she earned, by dint of association as a Singaporean and as her one-time friend.

Low noted that "there is a bit of Annabel in every Singaporean who dares to veer off the path well-trodden, and do something extraordinary with her or her life, not really caring about what people might think." Regardless of your stance on the way she did that, he concluded, "Annabel has imprinted herself firmly on our collective social consciousness" and he was writing that piece "to rehabilitate her within that social consciousness."

When I wrote to him in April 2007, it was to discuss his review of the stage play *251*, loosely based on the Annabel Chong legend, that had just run in Singapore. He wrote back:

Hi Gerrie

Thanks for your email and your very encouraging words. I sometimes wonder what Grace thinks of all the fuss around her and all that's been written about her, especially in Singapore. Please send my best regards to her as I haven't seen her in more than 15 years. We've both changed a lot since school and I really hope she is well and happy with her life.

I thought 251 was a play that used her story merely as a tool to drive home its own larger message about being different, censorship, repression, etc., and a lot of other angsty themes that are uniquely Singaporean. As a result, the character of Annabel Chong became a little too much of a caricature adapted to fit the plot and the message ... Still, I felt that I wanted to encourage the people who ultimately put the play up because I think the larger message is a sound one, especially in a closed-minded place like Singapore. And I think that a play about her is warranted for she really has made an impression (and not necessarily always a negative one) especially on our youth today and opened them up to more possibilities in life.

* * *

Ignatius Low's writing possessed an elegance that surpassed the previous time Annabel Chong made the local Singapore newspapers, in the *New Paper* "exposé" of January 27, 1997. The banner "EXCLUSIVE" was emblazoned on the paper's front page, followed by: "*Gifted S'pore student turns pornstar: The story she doesn't want told in Singapore, on Page 6*" with quotes taken from a telephone interview done with Annabel in Los Angeles.

The piece emphasized her squeaky-clean academic record – how she was in the gifted stream in a top school, had scored eight straight A's in her O-Levels, and was fondly remembered by her former teachers and classmates as "intelligent, sweet-looking and wholesome."

Then the reporter segues to January 22, 1995 and the big gangbang event because "she wanted to break the previous record (121 men)":

"I wanted to be the one to break the record first," she told The New Paper in a telephone interview from Los Angeles. At the time of her infamous sexploit, she had said: "People have called me a bimbo, slut and whore. But I enjoy my body. I enjoy sex."

Predictably, this *New Paper* piece ended on a moralistic tone, quoting a psychologist ("People with self-esteem will be concerned about what people think and perceive about them. Miss Chong may seem to be at ease with her actions but this is actually just an empty shell") and it also made note of the personal costs of her career, citing how she had lost friends she had grown up with and that "her former principals and teachers do not want to have anything to do with her."

So that's the *New Paper* perspective. Boo-hoo. Poor poor pitiful Annabel. This shunning of the black sheep only panders to the self-righteous folks out there, those who think that life is based on sets of absolutes. People who really believe that that everything has to be very black-and-white, and demarcated by the perimeters of their own conservative outlook.

But they've forgotten one thing: Life is often shades of gray, not always black-and-white, and things are sometimes not as infuriatingly simple as you would like them to be.

The sex industry is a good case study, since it's one of the most tangled webs I have seen people weave. Lots of flies get trapped for spider food, most vividly in the physical guise of chirpy young girls arriving by the busload (or, in Los Angeles, by carloads off the freeway) to the porn sound stages and production offices of the San Fernando Valley. Many of these impressionable young girls start out not entirely knowing what they're getting into. There's a difference, actually, between being a fish out of water and being in over your head, and sometimes it's hard to actually tell the difference.

But I enjoy the challenge of discerning that difference. And I'd submit that those ultra-conservative, judgemental people lack the mental agility to comprehend the complexities, so they merely wave it all off like pointless piffle. Also, it's an industry that doesn't exist in staid places like Singapore, so it's all too convenient to dismiss it as something mad, bad and dangerous to know. (The recent revolution in cellphone porn has begun to change that view, though, and I'm glad technology has given them something to think about now.)

Here's the most profound articulation of my own view, which comes from my friend Lily Burana and her memoir, *Strip City: A Stripper's Farewell Journey Across America*, published in 2001. There's a wonderfully touching section where she tells of her first stripping job, her initiation at Peepland in New York City, leading to this realization:

I know the threshold I have crossed, that I have entered a dangerous and possibly damaging world. This is not cosmetic defiance like being a hardcore kid; a very serious taboo has been broken, and there's no turning back. This is scary, but in a small, sleazy way, it's exciting, too. I would never have thought that I'd do something like this, but now that I have, I am full of my own daring. I feel more in control of my life than I have in months.

In my journal that night, I write with a flourish of neophyte brio, 'I am working this business, it's not working me,' not yet knowing that in this business everyone gets worked, at least a little bit.

Yes, everyone gets worked. Everyone. As much as you think you are empowering yourself, you are also exposing yourself, literally, to exploitation. Nobody who works in any aspect of the sex industry for any length of time would dispute that.

The ones that do just haven't been around long enough.

Annabel Chong worked the industry to her advantage by taking advantage of the collective avarice that enables something like a massive, record-breaking gangbang event to actually take place, with ancillary marketing and merchandising thrown in for good measure.

But the industry certainly worked her back, by empowering the likes of director John Bowen and producer Chuck Zane, who somehow "failed" to pay her for her ten-hour marathon.

And when their company Fantastic Pictures finally died, everything came full circle.

*   *   *

What fascinates me about the porn industry is the seemingly endless permutations of preferences, often translated into particular fetishes, because lots of people like lots of different things. It's one of the most democratic sub-genres of pop culture that has ever existed, because there is truly something for everyone.

As director Andrew Blake once told me, when I interviewed him about his style of high-end, fetish-fashion porn: "When people who are hungry want something to eat, there are people that will go to a beautiful restaurant and have a three hundred dollar meal. And there's going to be the other people, that are going to go down to McDonald's for some fries and a Big Mac. That's the difference – I'm the expensive restaurant."

Annabel Chong never worked with Andrew Blake. His kind of porn just wasn't her stock in trade. For some people, porn is the visual equivalent of the McDonald's, where it's fast and disposable, and those were the kind of movies that she made – cheap and cheerful, schlocky at worst, satirical at best. And there's nothing wrong with that. I might not choose to see it, but that's my own choice. She had lots of fans who did.

And by that kind of pluralistic yardstick, the "one size fits all" way of conformist thinking that people like Annabel and myself grew up with back in Singapore just didn't cut the mustard. The people who bought the propaganda of that antiquated system were the very people who would never have understood her or her kind anyway.

In the end, the resulting "Confucian confusion" (as I like to call it) merely fed a growing insurgency, an army of proxy Annabels who chose to vote with their feet like she did. It was a loss for such a young country; for the fact remains that someone as smart as Annabel had chosen to leave to find her true calling elsewhere – when she could just as easily have made truly great contributions to the country, had they provided her with an environment conducive to staying.

To me, however, the finest articulation of her status as a Singapore rebel came from some early drafts of text for her personal website. I remember she sent me a lovely autobiographical section called "Bye Bye Law School, Hello Art School," which explained a great deal about how she saw herself:

I dropped out of law school at King's College London in 1992 to study art. For a Singaporean girl, that is a totally unacceptable thing to do. For Lee Kuan Yew's sake, you are supposed to grow up to be a lawyer, an engineer or a doctor. When they found out, my parents' friends and relatives, bless their hearts, called my parents to offer their condolences. It's nice to have people care about you, isn't it? Heart-warming stuff, indeed.

I left King's College, UK, to go to the University of Southern California, US of A. USC was a bit of a fluke, actually. I was in the process of applying to UCLA when my mom gave me a call telling me she filled in an application for me, forged my signature, and guess what, darling, you got accepted! I was very astonished, as a year ago, when I quit Law School to take up the Fine Arts, my parents reacted by cutting off my finances. Apparently, she has not only come round, but also taken upon herself to support my cause.

I resisted her initially, as I was concerned that USC is the bastion of conservatism, and totally antithetical to my goals to get a liberal education, and I will be dealing with all these conservative assholes, yada yada yada. My mom is a tough broad. She stood her ground. After all she put herself through on my behalf to go through the laborious American university application process. "Do you think you are too chicken to deal with people who disagree with your point of view?" she demanded.

That was a direct challenge to my womanhood. After all, I come from a family of Tough Asian Broads, and it has been a family tradition ever since. After all, my grandma was the first woman in Singapore to resist getting her feet bound. My mom resisted a traditional arranged marriage by chasing the matchmaker out of the house with a large broom. I will be expected to tough it out in a 'conservative environment.'

I took her up on it.

Like she said, heart-warming stuff indeed. She had learned feminism from her mother, leaving the country but only to exchange one conservative environment for another. But it was a new environment that gave her the means to transcend the limitations of her Singapore roots, one that actually allowed her to thrive.

A rebel is not without honor, as the saying goes, except perhaps in her own country.

7

THE SAND MANDALA

So where did Annabel Chong go, beyond her proverbial fifteen minutes? Where does anyone go, really, after they've exhausted their ride of fame?

There are some, like Annabel, who make me recall the words of my friend Sherry Ziegelmeyer, an adult-industry publicist who has been in the business for many years and has certainly seen the girls all come and go. She concluded that some of them do leave the industry "fairly balanced and whole."

"That is the type of thing most people do not realize – our industry accepts everyone as they are," she told me. "Most broken people came into this business that way. This business didn't cause the breaking. A handful do break while working in adult, and usually it is because they shouldn't have been here in the first place. Some thrive here, others don't. The ones that don't usually aren't going to thrive anywhere else either."

Or, as my favorite director Andrew Blake once so wryly told me, "The girls all come and go. And some of them should go."

I think there's no better testimony of how Annabel left the adult film business ("fairly balanced and whole") than the way she dealt with her website. To me, the manner in which she built and then dismantled it resembled a Tibetan sand *mandala* – how Tibetan Buddhist monks would work so hard at creating sand paintings with the utmost care and diligence, only to finally destroy them as a reminder of the impermanence of things.

*   *   *

In 2007, Annabel introduced me to the person who was her creative partner on her site, a photographer in Los Angeles whom I'll call Lawrence (at his own request). He told me they'd first met at a strip club after he'd already started shooting pornstars for their personal websites, an idea inspired by Mimi Miyagi after he'd met her at one of her movie release parties. "This was back in 1998, when the Internet was just starting up," he recalled. "I had a lot of ideas about marketing for these websites and I told Annabel some of these ideas. Being well-educated, she started thinking about them too, and that's how we became friends.

"About a year or two later, she said to me: 'You know what, maybe we should start a website and see what happens.' So she became the web programmer and I took the pictures. We started with this fundamental principle: We'll take lots of photos, they don't need to be super-pretty, but we're going to focus on not just having nasty sex pictures. We're going to focus on 'getting to know Annabel Chong.' So I shot her and we launched her website together – *annabelchong.com*; she did the programming while I did the photography, she managed the merchant account and I worked on how the marketing would be done.

"She actually would write down her daily activities and I would tell her to write about what made her feel good or what made her feel bad. And don't talk about sex, necessarily. It was interesting because we noticed that people who went to the site usually started by going to the pictures and then they go to the diaries. After a while, we noticed they went straight to the diaries – they didn't even bother looking at the pictures. They go straight to the diaries or to the chatroom, and they would ask fairly mundane questions – "What kind of groceries do you like to shop for?" "What do you think is the best grocery chain?" "How do you get along with your parents?" Me and Annabel were going to create a second site, of other girls other than her, but she eventually transitioned away from the industry – Grace decided to drop out of the field."

Drop out she certainly did, when she announced her retirement and simultaneously pulled the plug on her site in 2003. For those who missed out on the all-too-brief run of *www.annabelchong.com*, I'm going to reiterate some of the more stellar items on the menu, simply because for all intents and purposes they comprise Annabel Chong's last will and testament.

It really was the very last thing she did in public view before "Annabel" vanished forever.

The site opened with a page that simply said: "About Me." It read like this:

Welcome to my excellent website!

Just like Asia Carrera's site, this is a complete DIY job. I went to school to learn web design and here are the results – I hope you like the site as much as I do. This has been a very hands-on experience for me, and I find it very satisfying. I like the fact that I am in control of the entire process, and can make this site the best ever. I spend a lot of time updating this site and I enjoy visiting my message board to chat with y'all.

Now a little bit more about me. I grew up in Singapore, and left home to pursue my education, first in England and then in the States. While in college, I took an interest in the adult film industry, and made a few movies for a lark. After that, I decided to get serious, completed my degree at USC, and worked for 2 years as a journalist. To supplement my income, I also worked as an exotic dancer. At the same time, I was also flying around the world promoting the documentary about my life, Sex: The Annabel Chong Story. All this traveling burned me out. I made enough money to buy a house, but I was perpetually jet-lagged and depressed. I decided to go back to school to study computer programming, web design and networking, so that I can make a living without dealing with airports!

As of right now, I spend most of my time working my real job as a web designer and computer programmer. In my free time, I play golf, hike, fish and shoot rifles. However, occasionally the weather gets pretty hot out here in Los Angeles, and so I feel a need to get naked. Oh, and the camera just happens to be there, by the way.

Thank you for visiting my site, and enjoy!

I loved how that opening page snaked its way from serious to playful, and that last bit of titillation was intentional since half the site was intended to be "academic" and the other half totally "adult" – that way, she told me, people could choose which Annabel Chong they wanted, the geeky computer nerd or the exhibitionistic porn chick. Both were part of her and she wasn't going to apologize for them.

I also noticed that the big gangbang event of 1995, the one that made her famous in the first place, was not mentioned at all. (She "made a few movies for a lark"? Talk about understatement!) Then there was a membership page, which began with a very fetching, pixie-faced photo of her with the slogan: "You are not alone."

JOIN ME!!! DON'T BE SHY!!! This is your opportunity to get to know me better. Not only will you be able to see more than 150 new photos every two weeks (thousands already), you will also be able to chat with me and your fellow members in my private chatroom. In a few months' time, you will get *to see video clips and play Flash games that are created by me exclusively for my website. I will also be interviewing your favorite adult stars fcr my site, and posting photos of my exciting encounters with them. What are you waiting for? Membership is only $19.95 per month, so click on the button below and join me now!*

One of the more fun parts of my discussions with her about her site dealt with the thing most people were willing to pay to see – the photos. This was initially sent to me as a page of instructions entitled PICTURES, with statements like: "I have arranged the photos into photo 'sets.' Each 'set' is divided into 2 phases. Phase 1 photos are in the top pocket of the sleeve (unless otherwise indicated). They are the 'teaser' photos. For now, you just need to concentrate on the Phase 1s. The Phase 2 photos are meant for members only. Membership is not available yet, but I am working on it."

This led to further instructions about how to view the photos, followed by some brief descriptions of the different photo 'sets' themselves. These included previously unpublished film stills, photos of her before she became "Annabel," nude photo shoots from her private archives, and photos of her very own good self playing with herself (using her dildo collection). There was also a rather painful one called "Bound and Pegged," demonstrating how she initiated a guy into BDSM (bondage-discipline/sadomasochism) by sticking ten clothes pins onto his erect penis.

Then, there was the "Merchandise" section, which was in development when we last spoke about it since she hadn't yet set up the e-commerce end of the site. But the idea was to sell a bunch of cool stuff such as autographed magazines and videos, photos exclusively available from this website, and her "personal souvenirs" including bras, panties, shoes, and other personal effects.

There was also the "News" page, filled with updates on recent developments – in the beginning of the year 2000, for instance, she announced the theatrical release of the *Sex: The Annabel Chong Story* documentary film, her strip club tour dates, her intentions to start a new production company in partnership with the director David Aaron Clark, and her plans to film a second documentary ("about what it is like to be a documentary film subject … a personal and at times humorous look at the foibles of self-promotion").

The second documentary film was eventually shelved, as was the new production company she was trying to form. (I seem to recall that the whole mess started when Impressive Productions underwent financial hiccups and finally folded.) The original idea was for her to direct a fetish line for Impressive and direct high-end features with David Aaron Clark for the new company, with "soft" versions for cable and "hard" versions for video. (David Aaron Clark died from a pulmonary embolism, in November 2009, one year short of his 50th birthday.)

The talk shows were being funded by her documentary producer David Whitten, under the aegis of his company Greycat Releasing. The original idea was to do three episodes at half-an-hour each. "School for Strippers" would be shot in Vancouver. There were plans to do spoofs like "Sex Cults" (about UFO abductions, among other things) and "The Secret Life of Jasmin St Claire" (exploring Jasmin's post-porn career on the pro-wrestling circuit), and a contest called "Win a Date with Annabel Chong."

Everything was timed to coincide with the theatrical release of *Sex: The Annabel Chong Story* in the theatres, opening February 11, 2000 at the Quad in New York City and February 25, 2000 at Laemmle's Sunset 5 cineplex on Sunset Boulevard in Los Angeles.

To her credit, the site chugged along nicely for a while, and I remember some hilarious bits and pieces. This was the pre-Twitter era – and "blogs" as we know them today hadn't even existed yet – but she was already getting the world ready for bite-size updates of her life.

Here are some of the more memorable ones:

5 July 2002: Yours truly has gone completely wireless with her home network. Yes! Now I can do my emails while taking a crap. In the eternal words of Martha Stewart: "This is a good thing." So here is what I have: 5 PCs, two of which are wireless, and one Mac, ALL FULLY NETWORKED. I feel like a civilized adult and a tech goddess, although, frankly speaking, installing a LAN is not brain surgery.

6 August 2002: Nose to the grindstone. I am beginning to dream in SQL, PL/SQL and C++ (I used to dream in HTML but I have evolved to a higher level of geekdom, see?) The life of ex-Pornstar Annabel Chong is indeed glamorous, no? That being said, I do have a photo shoot for an Asian Dreamgirls calendar this Thursday, so I will have to drag myself away from the computer and look pretty ... It will be nice to get in touch with my feminine side this Thursday.

11 August 2002: I had a really spicy curry last night, and today my butthole is on fire. ARRRGH! I can barely sit down, and I had to apply an ice cube onto my butthole just to cool it down. I regret telling the dude at the Indian joint: "Make it extra spicy."

12 August 2002: This is day 2 and my butthole is still burning from that curry. Arrrgh! I practically had to use a fire extinguisher to put out the flames.

13 August 2002: Success! I managed to do my you-know-what this morning without setting my butt on fire. (Very good.) I celebrated by having some very spicy tom yum soup. (Bad.) I told the dude at my local Thai place to make it extra spicy. (Very bad.) Hopefully I will not have to call the fire department tomorrow.

This was accompanied by color photos of her cats – Brando, Bo, Newt and Chicken. She could certainly be funnier than anyone might expect, at least in a droll and wry and subversively philosophical sort of way. There was even a section called "Chickens," where she talked about why she liked them:

I like chickens. I collect the damn things. Chickens seem to run all over the place for no apparent reason whatsoever, and that is very perplexing to me. I do not understand chickens at all, and they are the only thing I like that I could not completely rationalize. I mean, I like sex, Foucault, CNN and broccoli, and I could definitely explain to you the reasons I like them. However, I have absolutely no clue why I like chickens.

Have you ever stared into the eyes of a chicken in order to understand it? Have you ever had any success in comprehending its hermetic Otherness? It is very much like staring into the eyes of God. God is the Other. So are chickens.

Here is an inventory of my chicken collection. You are invited to send me chickens to add to this collection. I will send you a photo of my butt in return. Just include your mailing address, and I will despatch the above-mentioned unmentionable to you in a discreet brown envelope.

This kind of gonzo humor made perfect sense to all and sundry later on when she decided to kill her website and left a single personalized note on a single webpage as a reminder of what a dazzling wit she possessed, almost the postmodern reincarnation of Oscar Wilde on recreational drugs.

For those of you who missed it, the page was entitled: "Whatever happened to Annabel Chong?" (accompanied by an illustrated logo of a farmyard chicken) and here's all it had to say:

Where's Annabel?

Annabel is dead, and is now replaced full-time by her Evil Doppelganger, who is incredibly bored with the entire concept of Annabel, and would prefer to do something else for a change. From her shallow grave, Annabel would like to thank her fans for all their love and support all these years, and to let them know she will never forget them.

In that case, what is this Evil Doppelganger up to nowadays?

The ED is a diabolical yuppie who is working as a web developer and consultant. She specializes in ASP and .NET with C#, Database Development and also does web design. While the divine Ms Chong was busy doing her Annabel thang, the ED was surreptitiously going to computer boot camp to pick up some skills, so that she can permanently kill off Annabel Chong and begin her new life of peace and relative obscurity. Now she is making a pretty decent living being a horrible geek and all that, proving there are second chapters in American lives, to hell with F. Scott Fitzgerald.

I would like to buy an autographed copy of the documentary. Where do I go?

Easy.

Click here.

Whassup with that chicken?

Beats me. That has left everyone totally flummoxed.

The "click here" is a hotlink, which goes to a page that read like this:

Get a Personalized, Autographed Sex: The Annabel Chong Story DVD Now.

The DVD will be signed "by Annabel Chong" – who will be rousted from her shallow grave by the ED for this purpose.

Please indicate if you would want to get this item personalized.

Includes an autographed 8x10 signed by the Evil Doppelganger & the late Ms Chong.

$39.99 (includes shipping via USPS)

Make Payments with PayPal – it's fast, free and secure!

Seven years have since passed, and the same page and link are still online, available from her Wikipedia page (and listed as "Archive of her official site, May 2003"). The PayPal request button, incidentally, leads to a dead link.

And that's how the legend ends, perpetrated by the legend herself as a gigantic cosmic joke on those who dare venture forth in attempts to uncover the mysteries of her mythology. That single webpage was her way of warning everyone that to do so would be, as they say, "not a good idea."

Say what you will, but I say you've got to at least admire that.

* * *

Around the time of Annabel's official retirement in 2003, I read a news report about some guy who was obviously a Jenna Jameson fan. He had paid US$5,600 for the honor of a one-day job – to caddy for Jenna at a charity golf tournament. The *eBay* auction, which began at US$469, finally ended when this guy beat 77 other people, all dying to carry Jenna's golf bag for her at the Malibu Country Club course for the annual Skylar Neil Memorial Golf Tournament (hosted by Motley Crue singer Vince Neil, in honor of his daughter Skylar who had died from cancer).

Jenna pledged to donate every dollar to the Skylar Neil Foundation, which would then distribute the money to that year's charity of choice (that year's being the Lili Claire Foundation, a nonprofit organization for children born with neurogenetic birth disorders). "I was really excited to see that the bidding went as high as it did because all the money goes to a great charity," she said. "It will be nice to meet my new caddy and have a great day on the course, and of course I will win the tournament."

That, from "the woman who put the star in pornstar," as *Rolling Stone* magazine called her. Were there other ways for a guy to spend US$5,600? It was perhaps a strange way to spend money but surely less bizarre than the way Annabel once collected US$150 from an obviously obsessed fan.

"The guy wanted me to shit into a bag for US$150," she said. "So I went out and scooped up some dog shit and mailed it to him. He was completely ecstatic, thinking it was my shit! Actually, he wrote to me telling me he ate the shit and it was delicious."

That was back in 2002, eight years after she'd started out in the adult film industry and one year before she officially retired from the business. For her, I thought, that one might have been the final nail in the coffin of celebrity. What the heck do you do for an encore after a request like that?

That anecdote stood out because I had first mentioned it in my porn-biz memoir *In Lust We Trust*, in a chapter about Annabel Chong and Asian pornstars, and someone who'd read the book told me later that it was the one section of the book that he couldn't get out of his head.

"A good time is not worth having if you can't remember it," as the novelist Tim Sandlin once told me. And the thing to note about the mythology of Annabel Chong is that the things we take from her celebrityhood that are truly valuable are the things we need to remember.

Not the spectacle of the big gangbang or the media frenzy that came with it. Or even the documentary (and the media frenzy that came with it). People do remember the parts of the film that were poignant, like where her mother breaks down and tries to deal with her daughter being a pornstar. And where Grace herself, shed of the bravado of the Annabel persona, cries herself over her need to make reparations to her mother. Some remember the parts where she cuts herself with razor blades to deal with her own emotional numbness.

I myself like the section where she returns to the porn industry after a hiatus and is seen negotiating with director Rob Black about performing certain sex scenes beyond her comfort zone. Black, known as an extreme porn practitioner, favoring scenes of simulated rape and various kinds of sexual violence, is seen in the film as a tough negotiator, asking for "fist, piss and anal." (A man of what can only be called questionable scruples, as several of my own porn industry sources have concurred, he was eventually jailed on obscenity charges in 2009 along with his wife, the director/performer Lizzy Borden.) Annabel, shot in her bedroom while wearing hair rollers and a face mask, is seen spending quite some time on the phone with him, unwilling to give in easily.

In all fairness, any non-industry civilian might well ask, "What could be so risky for your sexual comfort zone after you've already done a gangbang?"

More pointedly, in an era where the Internet has, ironically, made it easier than ever to access adult content and thereby has also diminished its power to tease and titillate, what does the cultural significance of the pornstar mean anymore?

We know now what we didn't know then: Annabel Chong's historic 1995 gangbang actually symbolized the end of an era, when porn still possessed a certain innocence now sadly gone, as the gangbang genre led to the "gonzo" porn explosion of the late-90s and "reality porn" then became the desired norm, making her a forerunner of things to come, something we all know now but only with the wisdom of hindsight.

The "gangbang" scenario back then was porn decontextualized – it was out of the ordinary, and had the gee-whiz quotient of the reality television shows that would captivate people years later, things like *Fear Factor* and extreme makeover shows like MTV's *I Want A Famous Face*.

She did it, on a scale no one had dared attempt before. And it really didn't matter what else she did after that.

Because the damage had already been done.

It exerted an effect that she had probably not expected – it polarized people yet also drew people towards porn. It piqued our collective curiosity, even altering the mindset of those previously unwilling to explore what the genre could offer. And that's the most lasting impact of the Annabel Chong legacy.

Nothing further that I could say about this sounds any better than something once uttered to me by the great Nina Hartley, then in her seventeenth year as a pornstar when I interviewed her back in 2001.

"My longevity in this business is partly because I'm famous and popular, and partly because I'm a role model for women, for a way to have sex and not feel used and degraded," she told me during a break in filming, at a studio off Santa Monica Boulevard in Hollywood. "I'm a sexual creature and a sexual revolutionary. I like having sex with various people because it's so subversive and powerful and, at the same time, it's very fun."

"And, also, I like having sex in public without getting arrested," she quipped. "We are each responsible for our own pleasure in life."

That sense of responsibility was what Annabel Chong represented, and what we have been searching for.

The memory of pleasure lasts longer than the feeling of fame, so who cares where anybody has gone after a fifteen-year lapse, when there hasn't yet been a lapse of memory?

For she reminds us, in the end, that we are the very things that we remember.

And, in that light, I still treasure my fond memories of "Annabel" – for she is part of who I am, or rather much that I myself believe in. After all, her message made perfect sense to me the very first time. What we do not learn, as they say, we are doomed to repeat.

POSTSCRIPT

On October 31, 2011, I received a note from Grace Quek saying she had finally found the time to read this book.

I hadn't heard back from her in the six months since I'd sent it to her, after the original edition came out in Asia in April of 2011. It had apparently been lying on her bookshelf waiting for the right moment. This is what she said in her email, in its entirety:

Hi Gerrie

I finally decided to read the book that you wrote about my doppelganger – or at least parts of it. Thank you for giving me a fair shake! I will finish the book this weekend and let you know what I think.

I have to admit it was a somewhat surreal experience – it was like reading a book about someone else. You certainly made me sound more legendary than I actually am. I was reading the book in between trying to chop up some large onions for a curry dinner I was hosting. The onions hurt my eyes, so I took multiple breaks in between. I did not feel remotely legendary at that point, I can tell you that! But you can say I teared up while reading your book – just do not mention the onions, OK?

    Cheers
    Grace

Wow, I thought, she certainly hasn't lost her sense of humor! And it did feel rather rewarding, I must admit. There are surely biographers whose books never even get read by their subjects or, worse, are actually viewed with contempt for reasons amounting to (in some cases, quite understandably) invasion of privacy. I was so relieved to finally know that I hadn't been dumped into that category.

A few weeks later, on November 23, the eve of Thanksgiving 2011, I called her just to wish her a happy turkey day and to see if she'd finally finished reading it – she told me she had and she'd liked it. She'd even lent the book to a friend, who had also enjoyed it. We talked on the phone for almost two hours. "Thanks for giving me a fair shake," she repeated, adding that she was sorry it had taken her so long. "I wasn't ready for it, back in April, and I needed time to deal with Annabel again."

Revisiting ancient history wasn't something she much cared to do these days, so it was certainly something of an imposition on my part; now I could at least rest assured she didn't hate the book. However, I also explained to her that I was in the process of writing a Postscript chapter that would conclude the American edition, which would explain some of the excisions and deletions from the original manuscript.

"Write whatever you want, Gerrie, I trust you," she said, when I asked if she minded if I included verbatim the note she had sent me earlier. I am naturally touched by her trust in me – itself an amazing thing, given the complexity of the text already written – and so without further ado (and to imaginary drum rolls and canned applause), here's all I have left to say.

* * *

In the course of any book being published, including this one, deletions and incisions are always necessary since it is the editor's prerogative to tighten up the text. However, it did occur to me not long after it first came out in April 2011 that perhaps some readers of this 2012 American edition might enjoy knowing the juicy bits that were lost.

There were some minor cuts, which don't require much revisiting here. For example, in the final draft I myself excised a paragraph devoted to my own reaction to an article about Annabel Chong ("The Child Defiled" by Gary Morris, in Chapter 5) because in the end it seemed superfluous. There was also the occasional sleight of space (the infamous "scooping the dogshit" section in Chapter 7 originally appeared at the start of the book) and there were also things I myself finally edited out, like how I'd been "sworn to secrecy" about Annabel's stripping gigs (in Chapter 5) simply because I didn't want to unnecessarily tarnish the reputation of certain habitues of the strip-club subculture.

A more major deletion that occurred, for somewhat similar reasons (because I felt it necessary to protect Annabel) was a fascinating episode relating to a series of email exchanges between Annabel, Asia Carrera and myself back in February 2004.

Asia sent me a note telling me one of her fans had informed her about a website he had discovered on which some nosy person had apparently posted Grace Quek's California driver's license, containing her personal details including her home address.

"I know someone who can reach Annabel," Asia told the fan, and forwarded the note to me. "That's totally uncool of someone to violate her privacy like that."

So I forwarded Asia's note onward, and Grace sent a reply that I thought quite priceless:

I have a new Cali license now, so that one is old. Thank God! Actually, they got most of that info from my old website. Bizarre how one lives on in cyberspace.

It is so cool that Asia is looking out for me. Tell her thanks! I am curious whether many fans tried to invade my old place – hah hah. Let 'em deal with the hairy husband from Iowa. He has a rifle too.

The "hairy husband" was her real-life ex-husband – yes, the real Grace Quek is divorced – and that was one reason for the deletion. This being a book about the power of persona as defined by Annabel, the porn star (and therefore not really about Grace, the real person), I felt reluctant to divulge that morsel of information about her private life.

Well, that and the fact that the ex-husband might not take so kindly to being described as a hirsute gunslinger.

On that note, there was another section which I myself omitted, relating to an exchange of correspondence I had with Grace at that same juncture in early 2004, whereby I told her I was writing about her in one of my books:

I am mentioning you in passing in one of the chapters, by the way, as a famous person from Singapore – alongside Julia Nickson, Fann Wong and Vanessa-Mae. Of course, poor Fann has only one Jackie Chan movie to her credit ("Shanghai Knights") and doesn't really count, ha-ha. And Julia Nickson, well, does anybody remember "Rambo: First Blood, Part 2"?

The other sections that were eventually cut related to the subtext of the book itself – the socio-political backdrop of Grace Quek growing up in a place like Singapore and how her cultural conditioning had affected her, leading her to eventually create her Annabel Chong alter ego.

For instance, my editor (at Monsoon Books, for the original edition published in Asia) had objected to a section from the first interview I did with her (as reproduced verbatim in Chapter 3), which he wanted to (and finally did) delete. It was merely one paragraph, in which she stated her position on the Singapore government:

The government posits itself as a kind of father – the "father knows best" – and a lot of people do swallow that.

Singaporeans are being subjected to a constant stream of propaganda and it's very insidious. I remember going to those National Day Parades and, although I'm thinking, "Oh God, this is bullshit" when everybody is screaming, it's really hard not to join them. You get carried away by the moment and I'd find myself, like, cheering, going, "Rah, rah, Singapore," whatever. Like singing "We Are Singapore" – what a terrible song! And I'd go home and think, "Did I actually sing very loudly and very happily to that song, like an hour ago?" How strange! But that is the power of propaganda. And I guess living in Los Angeles gives me enough space to resist it.

Here, the word "insidious" became a point of contention since it implied a value judgment, and I could also imagine an objection to her describing it as "the power of propaganda."

As noted elsewhere for some years now, the Singapore government has made a perniciously persistent habit of taking to court various journalists and publishers for printing things it self-righteously defines as defamatory. This kind of paranoia inevitably leads to self-censorship, so I felt this editor was actually feeding the flame instead.

My exact response to his objection was simply this: "But I didn't say it, she did! And this has been published before – that section appeared in *BigO* magazine back in 1999. And nothing happened!"

I originally ended Chapter 6 with a section that was also excised, in which I noted how Annabel had made her own perspective on this situation resoundingly clear:

Annabel actually explained all this much better and more succinctly than me, in a 2002 American Independence Day note to her fans on her personal website:

"The 4th of July is coming around the corner and I have hung out my flag. I may not be an American citizen yet, but I am proud to be part of this great country and look forward to being one soon . . . I was born in Singapore, a peaceful and prosperous country of great beauty. Visitors have often commented on the cleanliness and orderliness of the city, the way everything works like a well-oiled machine. However, one of the compromises we had to make for our high standard of living is that we have to give up many of our freedoms. We do not have freedom of press, freedom of association and freedom of speech. We live under a one-party dictatorship, albeit a benevolent one. However, benevolence could be suffocating, especially if you could be thrown into jail without trial for expressing a dissenting opinion."

I then followed this with my own choice words:

In the end, the resulting "Confucian confusion" (as I like to call it) merely fed a growing insurgency, an army of proxy Annabel Chongs who chose to vote with their feet like she did. (At that juncture, it was estimated that 250,000 people had already emigrated from Singapore.) It was, arguably, "nation-

building" gone awry, amounting to a huge loss for such a young country; the fact remains that someone as smart as Annabel chose to leave to find her true calling elsewhere – when she could just as easily have made truly great contributions to the country, had they provided her with an environment conducive to staying.

The current prime minister, Lee Hsien Loong, admitted that he understood this, if only indirectly and in passing, when he once stated how it was his aim for Singapore to be a country that the young people of the future would willingly choose to live in. He'd realized, to his credit, that in the rush towards being seen as a real "First World country," they had committed an egregious disservice to themselves by losing many talented people.

There was now an ongoing debate in the country about the urgent need to import "foreign talent" but this was actually something self-inflicted which began when, all those years ago, they had pushed people like Annabel Chong away.

In the end, I replaced that chunk of text with another, quoting her directly from previously unpublished early drafts of text from her personal website, which she'd given me privy to:

I dropped out of law school at King's College London in 1992 to study art. For a Singaporean girl, that is a totally unacceptable thing to do. For Lee Kuan Yew's sake, you are supposed to grow up to be a lawyer, an engineer or a doctor.

When they found out, my parents' friends and relatives, bless their hearts, called my parents to offer their condolences. It's nice to have people care about you, isn't it? Heart-warming stuff, indeed.

And so, ultimately, I was upstaged by her own brilliant sarcasm. It really worked out for the best in the end. Sure, there are days when I do wish I'd been given a wider berth to breathe more room into the text – through the inclusion of the aforementioned sections – but I do maintain that the essence of the text is nevertheless intact.

And, more importantly, while the cuts were arguably judicious to a fault, they failed to undermine the very reason why Annabel Chong remains important as an example of modern celebrity branding, without which this book need never have been written in the first place. It is my best hope, with this American edition, that people outside Singapore will come to understand what she stood for and why I sought to demystify her legend.

I'd really like to thank Jennifer McCartney, my editor at Skyhorse Publishing in New York, for her unyielding faith in this book. And for granting me this opportunity to set the record straight, so that I might now forever hold my peace.

Gerrie Lim
December 12, 2011

ACKNOWLEDGMENTS

The seed for this project was planted back in 1999 by Alex Smithline, a literary agent I met with in New York, who first suggested to me the idea of a book about Annabel Chong. While I rejected it then, I believe it timely to thank him now, a whole twelve years later. All good things happen in their own time.

I am immensely grateful to Grace Quek, who told me she didn't care about Annabel Chong anymore but who finally agreed to read galley pages without officially endorsing this book. There is something to be said for the value of friendship over the years and across the miles. Too bad we never got to go to Iceland.

I am deeply thankful to some friends who read chapters while they were still works-in-progress and who took time to offer their comments: Fiona Pang, Jennifer Thym, Vivienne Yeo and Sonya Yeung. And a special word of appreciation to Sara Tang of Passionately Yours.

Also, for the roles they played in rendering form and

function to my text: Philip Cheah, Loretta Chen, Elaine Ee, Alyssa Farry, Christine Fugate, Colin Goh, Ben Harrison, Adrian Havas, Eric Khoo, Alexis Lee, Ignatius Low, Kate Mayor, Ong Soh Chin, Joanita Titan and David Whitten.

And my colleagues in the adult arena, for their quotable quotes: Juli Ashton, Andrew Blake, Lily Burana, Asia Carrera, Nina Hartley, Jenna Jameson, Sabrina Johnson, Katsuni, Jill Kelly, Dyanna Lauren, Rebecca Lord, Melissa Monet, Cheyenne Silver, Mika Tan, Inari Vachs and Sherry Ziegelmeyer.

And some notable writers, worthy of praise: Sheridan Prasso for *The Asian Mystique: Dragon Ladies, Geisha Girls* and *Our Fantasies of the Exotic Orient*, in my opinion still the best book written on the subject (and from which I have quoted, in Chapter Four) and Ronald Weitzer for *Sex For Sale: Prostitution, Pornography and the Sex Industry* (from which the quote from sociologist Sharon Abbott is taken, in Chapter Two). I am also indebted to Nic Kelman's *Girls*, from which I discovered a certain Latin translation (also in Chapter Two).

And two comrades in the porn trenches: the late David Aaron Clark and a cool cat named Lawrence.

And two exemplars of *eminence grise*: Chuck Palahniuk and Paul Theroux.

And my divine consort, my regally Royal Hotness: P.H.

The title of this book owes its inspiration to the Rosanna Arquette documentary film *Searching for Debra Winger*.

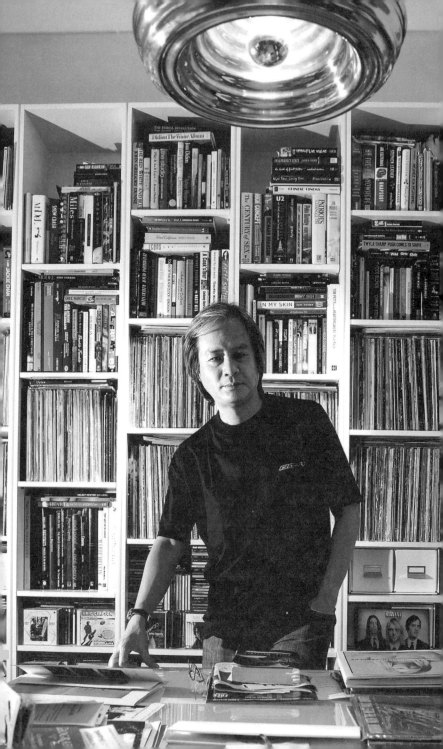